D0021435

FIT-OR-FAT
TARGET RECIPES

Soups

Salads

Sauces, Dips, and Dressings

Beef, Pork, and Veal

Poultry

Fish and Seafood

Beans and Other Legumes

Rice and Pasta

Vegetables

Breads

Desserts

Snacks and Beverages

FIT-OR-FAT®
TARGET RECIPES

Covert Bailey
and
Lea Bishop

Houghton Mifflin Company / Boston

For information about permission to reproduce selections from
this book, write to Permissions, Houghton Mifflin Company,
2 Park Street, Boston, Massachusetts 02108.

Library of Congress Cataloging in Publication Data
Bailey, Covert.
Target recipes.
Includes index.
1. Low-fat diet — Recipes. I. Bishop, Lea.
II. Title.
RM237.7.B35   1985   641.5′635   84-22365
ISBN 0-395-37698-X
ISBN 0-395-51084-8 (pbk.)

Printed in the United States of America

VB   15 14 13 12 11 10 9 8

Fit or Fat® is a registered trademark of Covert Bailey.

For
DORES BISHOP
and
BEE BAILEY
our testers and tasters —
Thank you, thank you,
thank you!!

Contents

The Fit-or-Fat System

AMERICANS EAT TOO MUCH FAT! Most people are surprised to learn that about 45 percent of the calories in their diet comes from fat. Even "health food" enthusiasts unknowingly eat an excess of high-fat foods. Fat contains few vitamins but lots of calories, making us nutrient-poor but calorie-rich.

In *The Fit-or-Fat Target Diet* foods are graded on a target, with low-fat foods at the center. As foods get progressively fattier, they are placed in rings farther from the bull's-eye.

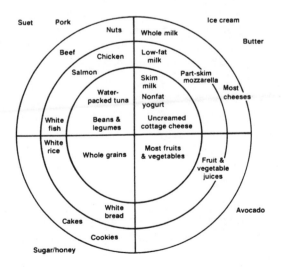

If you glance at the simplified version of the Target shown here, you may be shocked to find some of your favorite foods in the high-fat peripheral rings. You may also be surprised to learn that beef and peanuts have equally high fat levels, and beans and fish have equally low fat levels.

One gram of fat yields 9 calories, while 1 gram of carbohydrate yields only 4 calories. This fact should make it obvious that the fat in foods is what dramatically raises the calorie level, not the carbohydrate. Fats are fattening! Fat in the diet, coupled with a lack of exercise, is the principal cause of obesity, and obesity is our number one health problem. The single most overwhelmingly important dietary change people should make is to decrease their fat consumption. Some fat in the diet is recommended — in fact, essential — but we need to decrease our overall fat intake. The recipes in this book, in addition to being low in fat, follow all the other rules of good nutrition.

Low-fat, high-fiber cooking conjures up images of bland, unimaginative meals that are hard to swallow. When you try our recipes, you will be delighted! They are savory and totally satisfying, even to the most skeptical. You'll find low-fat cooking fun and challenging because it's hard to make food tasty without using butter and sugar.

Remember, everything in life is a compromise, and cooking is no exception. If you take *all* the sugar, fat, and salt out of foods, people won't eat them. Low fat doesn't mean no fat. People ask, "Don't we have to have *some* fat in the diet?" Of course we do. Glance at the recipes in this book, and you'll see that most have a little fat. We haven't cut out the fat, we've just reduced it.

So you will find some fat, sugar, and salt in most of our recipes, although in amounts lower than those in most cookbooks. Since the amount of fat is particularly critical, we show the fat content per serving for each recipe. We might have shown the grams of fat per serving, but used the term *fats* instead, to be in harmony with our background book *The Fit-or-Fat Target Diet.* By this system, 1 "fat" equals 5 grams or 45 calories. Look at the first recipe, for example, and you will see that one serving of Bailey's Bouillabaisse contains 130 calories and 1/10 "fat." Since each "fat" contains 45 calories, the 1/10 fat contributes 4½ calories to the serving; that is, 4½ of the 130 calories (about 3 percent) come from fat.

Although we didn't highlight sugar and salt content in the same manner as we did the fat, we have cut down on these ingredients, also. Readers of *Fit or Fat?* and *The Fit-or-Fat Target Diet* know we feel that fit people's bodies can handle sugar and salt much better than fat people's. But even if you're not fit you need not be concerned about our occasional use of ingredients that contain sugar, such as ketchup, or the modest amount of salt and bouillon cubes in the recipes. The quantities we suggest are below those recommended by the American Heart Association and are certainly safe for the average individual.

> We offer good home-style cooking with easy-to-follow directions. The recipes are simple and do not require unusual ingredients or trips to specialty stores. By following these recipes, even a novice can put together tasty, satisfying dishes.

Learn to Modify Recipes!

Many of the recipes in this book aren't "new" — they are simply modifications of older ones that call for too much fat or sugar. Don't feel that you have to throw away your old cookbooks or give up your favorite recipes. *Learn to change them.* It's not difficult. In many cases, we have included the original ingredients of recipes so you can see how we have changed them. Such modifications are so simple that making them will become second nature to you.

We urge you to make only small changes initially. Use low-fat milk instead of whole, substitute yogurt for sour cream, reduce the fats in recipes by a third. You'll be surprised at how little difference these small changes make in flavor. Pretty soon you won't depend on our cookbook because you'll be busy creating and experimenting with recipes all your own!

Recommended Daily Calorie and Fat Intake

We believe that everybody should have his or her percentage of body fat tested. We have written articles, newsletters, and even a book imploring people to have this test done. It is the only way to know for sure just how much fat your body has accumulated and the only rational way to decide how many calories you should eat. Nonetheless, we recognize that some readers haven't had their fat tested yet (hint, hint), and we have included a table, "Recommended Daily Calories and Fats," from which you can approximate your caloric needs. The easiest way to lower calories yet enjoy food is to restrict fat.

In this book we refer to the number of fats in a food: 1 fat equals 5 grams of fat equals 45 calories.

We expect most readers to fall into Category 2. Even if you are a Category 1 person, it is wise to stick to the low-fat recom-

Recommended Daily Calories and Fats

	If Your Percentage of Body Fat is		OR If You Don't Know Your Percentage of Body Fat* but You	You Should Eat			
				Calories/Day		Fats/Day	
	Men	Women		Men	Women	Men	Women
Cat. 1 (25% Fat Diet)	15% or less	22% or less	are satisfied with your present weight	2400– 2700	1700– 2000	No more than 15	No more than 11
Cat. 2 (20% Fat Diet)	16– 26%	23– 35%	want to lose 5–15 lbs.	1800– 2200	1400– 1700	8–10	6–8
Cat. 3 (10% Fat Diet)	27% or more	36% or more	want to lose more than 15 pounds	1400– 1800	1000– 1400	3–4	2–3

* *Caution:* Using weight as your criterion is not smart. Have your body fat tested, as above.

mendations of Category 2, knowing that you're allowed to "cheat" now and then. A Category 3 diet is very stringent and difficult to stick with. If you're quite obese or have had a heart attack, you *must* use this category. Category 3 is so strictly limiting that we have included a week's menus for you, to lessen the burden of getting started on it.

A few recipes in our book contain more fat than we normally recommend. These are for Category 1 people who exercise frequently. Their bodies burn fat well, so they can "afford" the extra fats.

Calories and Fats in Common Foods*

Meat Group

Quantity	Food	Calories	Fats
1 cup	Beans and other legumes	220	¼
3½ ounces	Beef (lean):		
	Tripe	155	½
	Heart	155	1
	Liver	155	1
	Top round steak	155	1
	Flank steak	155	1½
	Sirloin steak	155	1½
3½ ounces	Beef (moderately fatty):		
	Lean ground beef	200	2
	Lean chuck	200	2
	Club steak	200	2
	Bottom round steak	200	2
	T-bone steak	200	2
	Tenderloin steak	200	2
	Tongue	200	2
	Lean rib roast	200	2½
3½ ounces	Beef (fatty):		
	Cube steak	335	3
	Regular ground beef	335	3½
	Ground chuck	335	5
	Rump roast	335	5

* See *The Fit-or Fat Target Diet* for a complete list.

The Fit-or-Fat System

Quantity	Food	Calories	Fats
	Corned beef	335	6
	Rib roast	335	7½
	Rib eye steak	335	8
3½ ounces	Fish, all kinds except:	100	⅖†
	Mackerel	200	2
	Pompano	200	2
	Rainbow trout	200	2
	Salmon	235	3
3½ ounces	Lamb (lean)	155	1
3½ ounces	Lamb (lean and fat)	245	3
⅔ cup	Nuts and seeds	360†	5½†
3	Pork links	335	5
3½ ounces	Pork sausage	380	6
3½ ounces	Poultry, skinned white meat	130	⅔
3½ ounces	Poultry, skinned dark meat	155	1
3½ ounces	Poultry, with skin, dark or white	245	3
3½ ounces	Veal	155	1
2	Eggs	155	2

Milk Group

1 cup	Skim milk	90	0
	Buttermilk (made from skim)	90	0
	1% low-fat milk	100	½
	2% low-fat milk	120	1
	Whole milk	160	2
1⅓ ounces	Hard cheeses	110	2½
½ cup	Low-fat cottage cheese (uncreamed)	100	½
	Creamed cottage cheese	120	1
⅔ cup	Nonfat yogurt	90	0
	Plain low-fat yogurt	100	½

† Approximate quantity

Bread and Cereal Group

Quantity	Food	Calories	Fats
1 slice	White or whole-wheat bread	60	$^1\!/_{10}$
1 piece	Most cakes	160	2
1 ounce	Most cereals (sugar and fiber vary, but fat is usually low)	130	0
1 ounce	Chips:		
	Corn	160	2
	Potato and tortilla	160	1½
4	Most cookies	135	2
½ cup	Noodles, cooked	85	⅓
1 piece	Most pies	205	3
½ cup	Rice, white or brown	85	trace

Fruit and Vegetable Group

1 cup	Most vegetables	40	trace
1 cup	Most fruits except:	75	trace
½	Avocado	170	3½
6	Olives	110	2
½ cup	Fruit and vegetable juices	40	0

Menus for the Category 3 Diet Plan

(1000 to 1400 calories with 2 to 3 fats per day)

WE'VE DESIGNED a week's menus as a sample start for those of you who may require a very limited calorie/fat intake. We believe you'll be pleasantly surprised. You'll discover that by using these suggestions judiciously, you'll be able to enjoy a remarkable variety of foods in great quantities and remain within your calorie/fat restriction. There's no need to skip snacks. In fact, we urge you not to. If you find yourself eating five times a day, rejoice. You won't feel deprived because there's no reason to be. Conversely, don't feel that you've overeaten just because you are satisfied and hunger has vanished. We give you abundance, yet let you remain within the Target. These are delicious dishes — treats to your taste buds. You'll even be proud to serve them to guests.

This menu is also nutritionally well balanced. We have seen too many low-calorie, low-fat menus that are unbalanced, sometimes totally lacking in one or more food groups. With our plan, you will more than meet your daily vitamin/mineral and protein requirements.

> * Low-fat eating doesn't mean low quantity. In fact, some of you may find the daily menus simply *too* filling! Therefore, we have put asterisks next to the foods you can safely eliminate for that day without unbalancing the diet. *Caution:* If you do decide to eliminate some foods, be sure to tally up the total calories for the day. We urge you not to let your daily caloric intake go below 1000 calories. The metabolic consequences of fewer than 1000 calories a day aren't worth it. (For a more detailed explanation, refer to *The Fit-or-Fat Target Diet* by Covert Bailey.)

Daily Menus

Monday

Breakfast:	Cals.	Fats
½ grapefruit	40	0
1 Banana Raisin Muffin (see Breads)	160	1/5
1 cup skim milk	90	0
Coffee or tea	0	0

Snack:		
Apple-Flavored Yogurt (see Snacks and Beverages)	85	0

Lunch:		
Lentil Burgers with Dill Sauce (see Beans and Other Legumes)	248	½
Fresh pear or peach	75	0
Iced tea	0	0

Snack:		
Raw carrot*	40	0

Dinner:		
Fish Creole (see Fish and Seafood)	165	1/10
Cole Slaw with	40	0
Dressing (see Sauces, Dips, and Dressings)	28	0

Dinner (*cont.*)	Cals.	Fats
1 Corn on the Cob with Dressing (see Sauces,		
Dips, and Dressings)	127	$\frac{4}{5}$
Orange Pudding* (see Desserts)	80	$\frac{1}{2}$
	1178	$2\frac{1}{10}$

Tuesday

Breakfast:

1 poached egg	78	1
1 slice Oat-Wheat Bread, toasted (see		
Breads)	78	$\frac{1}{5}$
½ cup orange juice	40	0
Coffee or tea	0	0

Snack:

1 piece fresh fruit	75	0
1 Rolled-Oat Macaroon* (see Desserts)	53	$\frac{1}{5}$

Lunch:

Tuna Salad (see Fish and Seafood)	170	$\frac{2}{5}$
Tomato slices	40	0
1 cup skim milk	90	0

Snack:

1 slice Oat-Wheat Bread, toasted	78	$\frac{1}{5}$
1 slice Lite-line cheese	30	$\frac{1}{5}$

Dinner:

Chicken and Fresh Vegetables Provençale		
(see Poultry)	220	$\frac{3}{5}$
Curried Bean Sprout, Water Chestnut, and		
Fruit Salad (see Salads)	42	0
1 slice whole-wheat bread	60	$\frac{1}{10}$
Category 3 Custard with Egg Whites* (see		
Desserts)	87	0
1 Rolled-Oat Macaroon* (see Desserts)	53	$\frac{1}{5}$
	1194	$3\frac{1}{10}$

Wednesday

Breakfast:	Cals.	Fats
Hi-Fiber Lo-Fat Fruit Bran Milk Shake (see		
Snacks and Beverages)	180	⅕
Coffee or tea	0	0

Snack:		
½ cup fruit cocktail in water or light syrup	40	0
1 Rolled-Oat Macaroon* (see Desserts)	53	⅕

Lunch:		
Chili Bean Soup (see Soups)	245	¼
Whole-wheat pita pocket filled with	70	0
chopped vegetables and	40	0
2 tablespoons Yogurt Dressing (see Sauces,		
Dips, and Dressings)	20	⅒
1 cup skim milk	90	0

Snack:		
1 orange	75	0

Dinner:		
Savory Beef and Cabbage (see Beef, Pork,		
and Veal)	185	1½
½ cup noodles	85	⅓
½ cup Pickled Beets (see Salads)	75	0
1 Meringue Tart with Strawberries* (see		
Desserts)	122	0
	1280	2⅗

Thursday

Breakfast:		
2 pieces Quick French Toast (see Breads)	180	⅖
¼ cantaloupe	40	0
Coffee or tea	0	0

Snack:		
1 cup chicken bouillon	40	0
4 RyKrisp*	70	0

Lunch:	Cals.	Fats
White-meat chicken sandwich with	130	½
sliced tomatoes, lettuce, and	20	0
2 tablespoons Mayonnaise Substitute		
No. 1 (see Sauces, Dips, and Dressings)	8	0
on 2 slices whole-wheat bread	120	⅕
1 cup skim milk	90	0

Snack:		
Orange Cow (see Snacks and Beverages)	105	⅕

Dinner:		
Hearty Vegetable Soup (see Soups)	180	¼
2 slices whole-wheat bread*	120	⅕
Sliced pineapple with	40	0
½ cup low-fat cottage cheese	100	½
Buttermilk Sherbet* (see Desserts)	90	0
1 Rolled-Oat Macaroon* (see Desserts)	53	⅕
	1386	2½ (approx.)

Friday

Breakfast:		
2 shredded wheat biscuits	180	⅖
1 banana	75	0
1 cup skim milk	90	0
Coffee or tea	0	0

Snack:		
1 apple	75	0

Lunch:		
Split Pea and Barley Soup (see Soups)	275	⅖
1 slice Oat-Wheat Bread (see Breads)	78	⅕
Carrot and celery sticks, cherry tomatoes	40	0

Snack:		
Strawberry Yogurt (see Snacks and Beverages)	91	½

Dinner:		
Poached Sole with Cucumber Sauce (see Fish and Seafood)	96	⅕

Dinner (*cont.*)	Cals.	Fats
Fried Cabbage (see Vegetables)	42	3/5
Garden Pasta (see Rice and Pasta)	150	1/2
Angel food cake with raspberries*	140	0
	1332	2 4/5

Saturday

Breakfast:

2 Whole-Wheat Buckys (see Breads)	176	1 1/5
2 Turkey Sausages (see Poultry)	190	1
1/2 grapefruit	40	0
Coffee or tea	0	0

Snack:

1/2 cup tomato juice with celery stick	40	0

Lunch:

Lentil Curry Stew (see Beans and Other Legumes)	334	1/5
1 pear	75	0
1 cup skim milk	90	0

Snack:

Vanilla Delight (see Snacks and Beverages)	109	0

Dinner:

Broiled breast of chicken	130	1/2
Baked potato with	80	0
Mock Sour Cream* (see Sauces, Dips, and Dressings)	46	1/10
Tossed Salad with	40	0
French Dressing (see Sauces, Dips, and Dressings)	10	0
Quick Sherbet* (see Desserts)	50	0
	1410	3 (approx.)

Sunday

Breakfast:

Mock Soufflé (see Breads)	145	1
1 cup fresh fruit	75	0
Coffee or tea	0	0

Snack:	Cals.	Fats
4 RyKrisp	70	0
Carrot and celery sticks	20	0

Lunch:

Tuna sandwich (½ cup tuna) with	120	¼
lettuce and tomatoes and	20	0
2 tablespoons Mayonnaise Substitute		
No. 1 (see Sauces, Dips, and Dressings)	8	0
2 slices whole-wheat bread	120	⅕
1 cup skim milk	90	0

Snack:

2 cups popcorn lightly seasoned with garlic or celery salt (for the afternoon ball game!)	100	0

Dinner:

Veal and Lima Beans (see Beef, Pork, and Veal)	340	1
Eggplant Casserole (see Vegetables)	68	0
Cucumber Salad (see Salads)	30	1
Blueberry Bread Pudding* (see Desserts)	140	½
	1346	4 (approx.)

Soups

Zucchini Soup
(Serves 4)

With skim milk:
Calories per serving: 75
Fat per serving: trace

With low-fat yogurt:
Calories per serving: 92
Fat per serving: $\frac{1}{5}$

2 pounds zucchini, thinly sliced
1 cup chicken broth
1 cup diced onion
1 teaspoon curry powder

½ teaspoon salt
½ teaspoon pepper
1 cup skim milk or low-fat yogurt

Combine the zucchini, broth, onions, and seasonings and cook over medium-low heat until very tender. Put through a blender until smooth. Add the skim milk or yogurt. Adjust the seasoning. Serve hot or cold.

> When a recipe calls for the use of a blender, you can usually get the same results by using a food processor with a steel blade.

Bailey's Bouillabaisse (Fish Stew)
(Serves 9)

Calories per cup: 130
Fat per cup: $\frac{1}{10}$

1 large onion, diced
2 cups diced celery
3 small potatoes, diced
3 cups boiling water
2 cups skim milk
2 tablespoons flour
1 ½ pounds cod or flounder

2 cups diced broccoli
2 cups diced cauliflower
1 ½ teaspoons salt
½ teaspoon pepper
½ teaspoon marjoram
½ teaspoon basil

Cook the onion, celery, and potatoes in the water for 10 minutes. Mix a little milk with the flour to form a soupy paste and set aside. Add the remaining ingredients and bring to a boil. Add the flour mixture, stirring constantly. Simmer for 15 to 20 minutes.

Mushroom-Barley Soup
(Serves 8)

Calories per serving: 67
Fat per serving: trace

4 ounces fresh mushrooms,
    sliced
3 tablespoons pearl barley
2 quarts water
2 teaspoons salt

¼ teaspoon pepper
2 medium onions, diced
2 tablespoons flour
¾ cup skim milk

Combine the mushrooms, barley, water, salt, and pepper in a saucepan and cook over low heat for 1 hour. Brown the onions in a nonstick pan and add to the soup; cook for 30 minutes. Mix the flour with the milk and add to the soup. Cook for 15 minutes.

Curried Tuna Bisque
(Serves 4)

It's easy to modify a recipe! The original recipe calls for 2 tablespoons oil, whole milk, and oil-packed tuna. One serving contains 330 calories and 4 fats!

With skim milk:
Calories per serving: 200
Fat per serving: 1

With 2% low-fat milk:
Calories per serving: 220
Fats per serving: 1⅗

1 large carrot, shredded
1 medium onion, diced
1 medium celery stalk, diced
1 tablespoon salad oil
2 teaspoons curry powder
1 6½–7-ounce can water-packed tuna, drained and flaked
1 8¼-ounce can tomatoes

3½ cups skim or 2% low-fat milk
1 tablespoon cooking sherry or dry wine
1 chicken bouillon cube or envelope
2 tablespoons flour mixed with skim milk to form a soupy paste

Cook the carrot (except for 1 tablespoon), onions, and celery in the oil in a 4-quart saucepan over medium heat until tender, stirring occasionally. Stir in the curry powder; cook for 1 minute. Remove the pan from the heat; add the tuna and tomatoes with their liquid. Blend one-third of the tuna mixture in a blender at medium speed until very smooth; pour into a medium-sized bowl. Repeat with another third. Return the mixture to the saucepan with the remaining third and add the milk, sherry, bouillon, and flour. Boil for 1 minute to thicken, then reduce the heat and simmer for 5 minutes more. To serve, garnish the soup with the reserved shredded carrot.

Hearty Vegetable Soup
(Serves 10)

Calories per serving: 180
Fat per serving: ¼

2 16-ounce cans tomatoes, cut up
1 15½-ounce can red kidney beans
1 15-ounce can great northern beans
1 15-ounce can garbanzo beans
½ cup water
3 medium onions, chopped (1½ cups)

2 medium green peppers, chopped (1½ cups)
2 stalks celery, sliced (1 cup)
1 medium zucchini, halved lengthwise and sliced
2 cloves garlic, minced
2 teaspoons chili powder
1½ teaspoons dried basil, crushed
¼ teaspoon pepper
1 bay leaf

Combine the undrained tomatoes, undrained beans, water, and remaining vegetables and seasonings in a 4-quart Dutch-oven. Bring to a boil. Reduce the heat; cover and simmer for about 1 hour or until the vegetables are tender.

Light Minestrone
(Serves 8)

Calories per serving: 146
Fat per serving: ½

½ medium cabbage, coarsely chopped
1 medium onion, coarsely chopped
¼ cup chopped parsley
¼ teaspoon garlic powder
1 teaspoon oregano
½ teaspoon pepper

1 tablespoon oil
5 cups water
5 beef bouillon cubes
1 16-ounce can tomatoes
¼ pound spaghetti, broken up
1 medium zucchini, sliced
1 16-ounce can red kidney beans

Sauté the cabbage, onion, parsley, garlic powder, oregano, and pepper in the oil in a large pot for 5 minutes, stirring often. Add the water, bouillon cubes, and tomatoes. Bring to a boil. Stir in the spaghetti, zucchini, and beans. Cook for 10 minutes, stirring occasionally, or until the spaghetti is done.

Bean Soup
(Serves 4)

One of our readers sent us a "starter kit" for this recipe. It was a little bag containing every legume you can imagine — pinto, navy, green split pea, yellow pea, barley, kidney — you name it! Use your imagination and make up your own batch.

Calories per serving: 250
Fat per serving: $\frac{1}{5}$

1¼ cups dried legumes (use 10 to 12 different kinds)
¼ teaspoon ginger
1 large onion, chopped
¼ teaspoon lemon pepper
1 tablespoon barbecue sauce
½ teaspoon crushed red pepper pods *or* 1 teaspoon chopped green chili

1 small clove garlic, chopped
1 16-ounce can tomatoes
½ teaspoon chili powder
2 tablespoons ketchup
2 stalks celery, chopped

Wash the beans thoroughly. Place them in a large kettle and cover with 6 cups of cold water. Soak overnight. In the morning, without draining, add the ginger. Bring to a boil and cook until the mixture is tender. Add the remaining ingredients. Bring to a boil, then cut the heat and simmer for 2½ to 3 hours. Stir and add water as needed. (This is a great food to cook in a crockpot. After the first process, put everything in the pot, cook on high for 10 to 15 minutes, then on low for 5 to 6 hours.)

Country Kitchen Soup
(Serves 8)

Calories per serving: 190
Fat per serving: $\frac{1}{5}$

¼ cup baby lima beans
¼ cup small red beans
¼ cup yellow split peas
¼ cup green split peas
¼ cup lentils
¼ cup pinto beans
¼ cup pearl barley
2 quarts water

1 large ham bone
1 large onion, chopped
1 teaspoon chili powder
Salt and pepper to taste
2 tablespoons lemon juice
2 16-ounce cans tomatoes,
   chopped

Wash the beans and other legumes. Cover with cold water and soak overnight. Drain and add the water and ham bone. Bring to a boil and simmer for 2½ hours. Then add the remaining ingredients and simmer for at least 30 minutes more.

Pennsylvania Dutch Chicken and Corn Soup
(Serves 6)

Before we modified this recipe by skinning the chicken, it had 430 calories and 3 fats per serving.

Calories per serving: 290
Fat per serving: 1

3 whole chicken breasts,
   skinned and split
1 large onion, chopped
8 cups water
½ teaspoon salt
¼ teaspoon pepper
1 10-ounce package frozen
   whole-kernel corn

1 10-ounce package frozen
   chopped broccoli
1 cup all-purpose flour
1 tablespoon milk, low-fat or
   skim
1 egg

Place the chicken, breast side down, in a Dutch oven or large saucepan; add the onion, water, salt, and pepper. Heat to boiling; reduce heat, cover, and simmer for 35 minutes or until the chicken is tender. Let the chicken cool, remove the meat from the bones, and cut it into bite-sized pieces. Skim off the fat from the broth and heat the broth to boiling. Add the chicken, corn, and broccoli. Reheat to boiling. Meanwhile, mix the flour, milk, and egg in a small bowl with a fork. With your fingers, crumble small pieces of the dough mixture into the simmering soup; reduce the heat to medium; cook, uncovered, for 5 minutes or until the drops of dough and vegetables are tender.

Chili-Bean Soup
(Serves 4)

Calories per serving: 245
Fat per serving: ¼

1 medium onion, chopped fine
3 tablespoons water
1 28-ounce can kidney or pinto beans
1 28-ounce can tomatoes

1 6-ounce can tomato paste
1 tablespoon chili powder
½ tablespoon ground cumin

Slowly sauté the onion in the water in a 2-quart nonstick saucepan. Put the tomatoes in a blender and process for 30 seconds. Remove from the blender. Put the beans in the blender and blend for 30 seconds or until they have a lumpy consistency. Add the beans and tomatoes to the onions. Add the tomato paste and mix well. Add the chili powder and cumin and mix well. Bring the mixture to a boil, then reduce the heat and simmer for 30 minutes. The soup is best when it is prepared a day ahead, refrigerated overnight, and reheated.

Cold Tomato Herb Soup
(Serves 6)

Calories per serving: 50
Fat per serving: trace

2 beef bouillon cubes
1 cup boiling water
3 cups tomato or V-8 juice
1 small onion, grated
1 cup chopped celery
1 green pepper, minced
½ teaspoon salt

1 clove garlic
3 tablespoons lemon juice
Dash hot pepper sauce
2 tablespoons dried basil
1 cucumber, diced
2 ripe tomatoes, peeled and
    diced

Dissolve the bouillon cubes in the water. Cool slightly. Add the next five ingredients. Cut the garlic in half and stick a toothpick through both halves. Add to the mixture. Mix and refrigerate for several hours. Just before serving, remove the garlic and add the remaining ingredients. Serve cold.

Homemade Chicken Noodle Soup
(Serves 10)

This is Covert's favorite!

Calories per serving: 160
Fat per serving: ⅖

12 cups water
2 whole chicken breasts,
    skinned and split
2 stalks celery with leaves,
    chopped
6–7 green onions (scallions)
    with stems and tops, chopped

1 large onion, chopped
2 medium carrots, sliced
3 cups cooked egg noodles
1 cup plain low-fat yogurt

Place all the ingredients except the noodles and yogurt in a large pot and bring to a boil. Reduce the heat, cover, and simmer for 2 to 3 hours or until the chicken is tender. Add more water if necessary. Remove the chicken from the bones and cut it into bite-sized pieces. Return the chicken to the pot, along with the noodles. Simmer for 20 to 30 minutes so the noodles absorb the flavor of the chicken. Remove from the heat. Stir in the yogurt until thoroughly blended and serve.

In some areas green onions are better known as scallions.

Rishta (Lentil and Spinach Soup)
(Serves 6)

Calories per serving: 100
Fat per serving: ½

1 cup lentils	2 cups chopped fresh spinach
4 cups water	Salt and pepper to taste
1 large onion, chopped	1 cup dry noodles
1 tablespoon vegetable oil	Juice of 1 lemon (optional)

Wash the lentils and pick them clean. Combine the lentils and water in a saucepan and cook for 15 minutes. In the meantime, sauté the onion in the oil until light brown and add to the lentils. Add the spinach, salt, pepper, and noodles. Cook for 15 minutes. Add more water if necessary. Add the lemon juice and serve.

Split-Pea and Barley Soup
(Serves 8)

Calories per serving: 275
Fat per serving: ⅖

2 ham hocks   1 cup shredded carrot
2 cups split peas   1 large onion, diced
½ cup barley   ½ teaspoon salt
8 cups boiling water   ¼ teaspoon pepper
1 cup diced celery

Simmer the ham hocks, split peas, and barley in the boiling
water for 45 minutes. Take out the bones and trim the fat well,
returning the meat to the pot. Add the remaining ingredients
and simmer for another 45 minutes, adding water if the soup
gets too thick.

Turkey Chowder
(Serves 6)

Calories per serving: 144
Fat per serving: ½

1 medium onion, chopped   ½ teaspoon pepper
Turkey carcass   3 cups skim milk
4 cups boiling water   1½ cups (or more) cooked
1½ teaspoons salt   brown rice

Cook the onion in a nonstick pan or microwave oven until
tender. Break up the carcass and put it in the pan along with
the water, salt, and pepper. Add the onions. Cover, heat to
boiling, then simmer for 30 minutes. Remove the bones, scrape
off the meat, and add it to the soup. Add the milk and rice (or
noodles) and season to taste (poultry seasoning works beauti-
fully).

Hot and Sour Soup
(Serves 8)

Calories per serving: 230
Fat per serving: 1

4 whole medium chicken breasts, skinned, boned, and split
4 tablespoons soy sauce
1 tablespoon salad oil
6 cups water
½ to ¾ teaspoon finely ground white pepper
3 tablespoons white wine vinegar
¼ pound Chinese pea pods
1 medium red pepper, cut into thin strips
1 8-ounce can bamboo shoots, drained
2 chicken bouillon cubes
1 pound firm tofu (soybean curd), cut into bite-sized pieces
⅓ cup cornstarch
2 eggs
1 large green onion, thinly sliced

Cut the chicken into ⅛-inch slices. Stir the chicken slices with 1 tablespoon soy sauce in a bowl. Cook the chicken in the oil in a 5-quart Dutch oven until tender — about 3 minutes. Remove the chicken from the pan, add the remaining soy sauce to the pan along with the next seven ingredients, and heat to boiling, stirring frequently. Reduce the heat to low and simmer for about 10 minutes or until the vegetables are tender. Add the chicken and tofu and bring to a boil over medium heat. Stir the cornstarch and ⅓ cup of water in a small bowl until smooth. Gradually add the mixture to the simmering soup until slightly thickened and smooth. Beat the eggs in a small bowl and slowly pour them into the soup, stirring gently until they are set. Sprinkle the green onion over the soup.

> We often use nonfat dry instead of liquid milk in recipes: ⅓ cup nonfat dry milk plus ¾ cup water equals 1 cup liquid milk.

Salads

Brown Rice and Chicken Salad
with Wine Dressing
(Serves 4)

Calories per serving: 222
Fat per serving: 4/5

½ cup brown rice
1 cup water
¼ teaspoon salt
2 cups skinned and cooked
   cubed chicken

1 stalk celery, chopped
¼ cup chopped parsley
¼ cup sliced green onions
1 teaspoon dill weed
Wine Dressing (recipe follows)

Cook the rice in the water and salt as directed on the package. Drain. Combine the rice, chicken, celery, parsley, onions, and dill weed. Add as much dressing as desired. Toss.

Wine Dressing

1 cup low-fat cottage cheese
2 tablespoons wine vinegar
½ teaspoon pepper

¼ cup water
¼ teaspoon salt
1 ½ teaspoons mustard

Put all the ingredients into a blender and flash blend, by quickly turning the motor on and off. You will probably use about half the amount you made on the chicken salad.

Curried Bean Sprout, Water Chestnut, and Fruit Salad
(Serves 6)

This is an unusual salad — visually and for the palate.

Calories per serving: 42
Fat per serving: trace

2 cups fresh bean sprouts
¼ cup sliced water chestnuts
½ cup sliced seedless grapes
1 large peach, diced

¼ cup diced green pepper
¼ cup plain low-fat yogurt
1 teaspoon curry powder
1 teaspoon soy sauce

Combine the first five ingredients. Mix the yogurt, curry powder, and soy sauce together, and pour the dressing over the salad. Toss and serve.

All-American Low-Fat Potato Salad
(Serves 4)

Calories per serving: 130
Fat per serving: ⅕

3 medium potatoes, cooked,
   peeled, and cubed
5 green onions, sliced
2 stalks celery, diced
6 radishes, sliced (optional)

1 teaspoon dill weed
1 cup Yogurt Dressing (see
   Sauces, Dips, and Dressings)
1 cup diced cucumber

Combine the vegetables. Add the dill weed to the Yogurt Dressing and mix thoroughly with the salad. Refrigerate for several hours. Add the cucumber, toss all together gently, and refrigerate for 30 minutes before serving.

Put a feather in his hat and called it —

Yankee Doodle Macaroni Salad
(Serves 4)

Calories per serving: 138
Fat per serving: $\frac{1}{10}$

2 cups cooked salad macaroni
1 cup diced celery
1 cup grated carrot
½ cup diced green pepper
   (optional)

4 green onions, diced
Salt and pepper to taste

Mix the ingredients thoroughly with:

1 tablespoon prepared mustard
½ cup Mayonnaise Substitute
   No. 1 (see Sauces, Dips, and
   Dressings)

Cucumber Salad
(Serves 4)

Calories per serving: 30
Fat per serving: trace

½ teaspoon crushed dried mint
4 green onions, thinly sliced
   (optional)
½ cup Mock Sour Cream No. 2
   (see Sauces, Dips, and Dressings)

2 cucumbers, peeled, cut into
   crosswise slices, and chilled

Combine the mint and green onions with the Mock Sour Cream and pour over the cucumbers. Refrigerate before serving.

Bean Salad Bowl
(Serves 6)

Calories per serving: 123
Fat per serving: ⅕

1 16-ounce can cut green
  beans, drained
1 16-ounce can cut wax beans,
  drained
1 16-ounce can red kidney
  beans, drained
½ cup chopped onion (or use
  little green onions)

1 medium green pepper,
  slivered
1 cup plain low-fat yogurt
¼ teaspoon Worcestershire
  sauce
½ teaspoon garlic salt
1 teaspoon pickle relish

Toss the beans, onion, and pepper in a large bowl. Combine
the rest of the ingredients and pour over the beans. Refrigerate
for 3 hours, stirring frequently.

And Another Bean Salad . . .
(Serves 10)

We debated whether to use this recipe sent in by a reader, be-
cause the sugar content is a little high. But the original recipe had
3 cups of sugar. We think this one is a delicious modification!

Calories per serving: 313
Fat per serving: ⅖

1 cup sugar
½ teaspoon salt
1 cup vinegar
1 16-ounce can green beans,
  drained
1 16-ounce can yellow beans,
  drained
1 16-ounce can lima beans,
  drained

1 16-ounce can garbanzo
  beans, drained
1 16-ounce can red kidney
  beans, drained
1 green pepper, slivered
4 stalks celery, sliced
3 medium onions, sliced very
  thin

Combine the first three ingredients in a saucepan and bring to a boil; boil for 1 minute. Cool. Toss all the other ingredients together and pour the vinegar mixture over them. Marinate for 24 hours in the refrigerator, stirring occasionally.

String Bean Salad
(Serves 4)

Calories per serving: 25
Fat per serving: trace

1 16-ounce can (or fresh-cooked) string beans, drained
1 tablespoon chopped pimiento
½ cup French Dressing (see Sauces, Dips, and Dressings)

Chopped chives, chopped onion, or pearl onions

Marinate the beans and pimiento in the French Dressing for at least 3 hours, then add the onions. Chill thoroughly and serve on lettuce.

Spinach Salad
(Serves 4)

Calories per serving: 87
Fat per serving: ⅗

4 cups washed, dried, and chilled fresh spinach
1 cup sliced fresh mushrooms
4 radishes, sliced
1 tablespoon ketchup

1 teaspoon mustard
½ cup Mayonnaise Substitute No. 2 (see Sauces, Dips, and Dressings)

Combine the vegetables. Add the ketchup and mustard to the Mayonnaise Substitute and toss all together.

Mixed Vegetable Salad

Actually, you can use any fresh vegetables!

Calories per serving: 40
Fat per serving: trace

Cauliflower
Broccoli
Carrots
Celery

Mushrooms
Cherry tomatoes
Low-calorie, low-fat salad dress-
  ing of your choice*

Cut all the vegetables into small pieces. Marinate in the dressing for at least 8 hours.

Pickled-Beet Salad
(Serves 4)

Calories per serving: 75
Fat per serving: trace

1 16-ounce can beets, sliced
½ cup beet juice
½ cup white or wine vinegar
2 tablespoons sugar
½ teaspoon salt
1 ¼ bay leaf

½ green pepper, sliced
  (optional)
2 cloves
3 peppercorns
1 small onion, sliced

Boil the beet juice and vinegar. Add the remaining ingredients.
When the mixture returns to a boil, pour it over the beets.
Cover and chill for several hours.

* Refer to Sauces, Dips, and Dressings for lots of low-calorie dressings. Or simply use an instant salad dressing to which you add just water and vinegar — *No
oil!!*

Hot Potato and Broccoli Salad
(Serves 6)

This is a delicious salad, but use it sparingly if you have to limit your daily fats.

Calories per serving: 160
Fats per serving: 2

4 medium potatoes, peeled
1 bunch broccoli, trimmed and
  broken into small florets
¼ cup vegetable or salad oil
¼ cup lemon juice
¼ teaspoon garlic powder

¾ teaspoon salt
1 teaspoon basil
¼ teaspoon liquid hot pepper
  sauce
2 green onions (scallions) with
  stems, sliced

Cook the potatoes until tender, then dice them; cook the broccoli until tender. Keep both hot. Combine the remaining ingredients. Bring just to a boil, stirring. Pour over the vegetables and toss gently. This salad is also delicious served cold.

- Add leftover vegetables to salads rather than re-heating them.
- Last night's salad will stay crisp for today's lunch if you store it in an airtight container. Add a thermos of hot soup, some whole-wheat bread, and enjoy your lunch hour in the park instead of a noisy restaurant.

Sauces, Dips, and Dressings

We've given extra-thoughtful attention to our salad dressings. It was no easy task, but we made several breakthroughs. Mindful of the 100 calories in a tablespoon of mayonnaise and 70 to 100 in the same amount of regular dressings, we succeeded in providing you with a wide choice of concoctions, quickly and easily prepared, with fewer than 20 calories per tablespoon.

Quick Tomato Sauce
(Makes about 3½ cups)

Calories per ¼ cup: 10
Fat per ¼ cup: trace

½ cup chopped onion
½ cup chicken bouillon
3 cups coarsely chopped tomatoes
1 teaspoon frozen apple juice concentrate

½ teaspoon oregano
½ teaspoon thyme
½ teaspoon basil
1 teaspoon garlic powder
Pepper

Cook the onions in the bouillon until soft. Add the remaining ingredients. Bring to a boil, cover, and simmer for 30 to 45 minutes.

Cream Sauce No. 1

Calories per ¼ cup: 50
Fat per ¼ cup: trace

2 cups skim milk   Salt and pepper to taste
1 tablespoon arrowroot
2 tablespoons chicken stock or
  bouillon

Stir all the ingredients over low heat with a wire whisk until
the sauce thickens — about 15 minutes. This is a good base for
a curry sauce.

Cream Sauce No. 2

Calories per ¼ cup: 31
Fat per ¼ cup: trace

1 tablespoon cornstarch   Salt and pepper to taste
1 cup skim milk

Cook the cornstarch and milk over low heat until the sauce
thickens. Season with the salt and pepper. Add to leftover
meats or vegetables.

Mock Sour Cream No. 1

Calories per ¼ cup: 50
Fat per ¼ cup: ¼

1 cup low-fat cottage cheese   Minced parsley
1 teaspoon prepared horseradish

Purée the cheese in a blender and combine it and the horseradish in a small bowl. Garnish with minced parsley.

Mock Sour Cream No. 2

Calories per ¼ cup: 46
Fat per ¼ cup: ¹⁄₁₀

¼ cup water *or* skim milk
1 cup low-fat cottage cheese

1 tablespoon lemon juice
⅛ teaspoon salt

Put all the ingredients into a blender. Process for 30 seconds.
Flash blend until creamy.

*Both these recipes can be used in place of regular sour cream,
which contains 104 calories and 2 fats per ¼ cup.*

About salt:

As a good rule of thumb, allow no more than ⅛ teaspoon salt per serving. For example, if a recipe
makes 4 servings, use no more than ½ teaspoon
salt (⅛ × 4 = ½).

Tuna Dip
(Makes 2 cups)

Calories per ¼ cup: 53
Fat per ¼ cup: ⅕

1 cup low-fat cottage cheese
1 6- or 7-ounce can water-
  packed white tuna

2 teaspoons grated onion
2 tablespoons chopped pimiento
Salt and pepper to taste

Process the cottage cheese in a blender or electric mixer at high
speed until it is smooth and soft. Drain and flake the tuna and
combine it with the cottage cheese, onion, pimiento, and seasoning.

Spinach and Herb Dip for Raw Vegetables
(Makes 4 cups)

Calories per ¼ cup: 31
Fat per ¼ cup: ¹⁄₁₀

3 cups plain nonfat yogurt
1 cup chopped spinach
½ cup chopped parsley
½ cup chopped chives

¼ cup chopped dill
1 clove garlic, pressed
Salt to taste

Combine all the ingredients. Chill for at least 3 hours.

Use fresh raw vegetables with your dips. If you prefer crackers, stick with the whole-wheat or whole-rye varieties such as RyKrisp, rice cakes, matzo, or wheat wafers. Get used to reading labels. Buy crackers that list *whole* wheat or *whole* rye as the first item on the ingredient list. If the first ingredient is enriched wheat flour, it's *not* whole wheat.

Tofu Dip
(Makes 2 cups)

Calories per ¼ cup: 32
Fat per ¼ cup: ¹⁄₅

1 cup mashed tofu
1 clove garlic, minced
½ cup finely chopped green
   onions

1 teaspoon chopped parsley
½ cup plain low-fat yogurt
1 teaspoon Dijon mustard
Pepper

Place all the ingredients in a blender and process for 30 seconds. Chill for several hours.

Bean Dip
(Makes 2 cups)

Bean dips are good with cut-up raw vegetables or as spreads for sandwiches.

Calories per ¼ cup: 74
Fat per ¼ cup: trace

2 cups cooked pinto beans
½ teaspoon garlic powder
2 tablespoons diced green
  chilies

1 teaspoon Dijon mustard
2 teaspoons cider vinegar
2 tablespoons chopped parsley
2 to 3 drops Tabasco sauce

Combine all the ingredients in a blender. Process until thoroughly mixed. Chill for several hours. Garnish with chopped chives.

Red Bean Dip
(Makes 1 cup)

Calories per ¼ cup: 60
Fat per ¼ cup: trace

1 15-ounce can red beans,
  drained (save the juice)
¼ cup red bean juice
½ cup chopped onion

1 large clove garlic
¼ teaspoon salt
¼ teaspoon cumin
Dash Tabasco sauce

Process the ingredients in a blender. Heat and serve with low-fat crackers.

Low-Calorie Dip
(Makes 1½ cups)

Calories per ¼ cup: 40
Fat per ¼ cup: ⅕

½ cup plain low-fat yogurt
1 cup low-fat cottage cheese
3 tablespoons chopped chives
2 tablespoons chopped parsley
1 clove garlic, crushed

½ teaspoon salt
1 teaspoon Worcestershire
  sauce
¼ teaspoon red pepper sauce

Put all the ingredients in a blender and process until smooth.
Refrigerate for at least 2 hours.

Celery Seed Dressing
(Makes about 2 cups)

We eliminated the oil (1 cup) and salt (1 teaspoon) from the original recipe and reduced the calories from 80 to 10, and the fats from 1½ to just a trace, per tablespoon.

Calories per ¼ cup: 43
Calories per tablespoon: 10
Fat: trace

½ cup confectioners' sugar
¼ cup apple cider vinegar
2 teaspoons prepared mustard

1 teaspoon paprika
1 teaspoon celery seed
1 cup water

Mix all the ingredients and shake well.

Dressing for Corn on the Cob
(Serves 4)

Although we use some butter in this dressing, it takes only 1 tablespoon for four ears. The other ingredients stretch the butter and add a delightful flavor to the corn.

Calories per cob with dressing: 127
Fat per cob with dressing: $^4/_5$

1 tablespoon margarine or butter
1 tablespoon prepared mustard
1 teaspoon seasoned salt

½ teaspoon pepper
1 tablespoon chopped fresh
  parsley

Blend all the ingredients together with a fork on a flat platter. Store in the refrigerator until the corn is cooked and ready to serve. Put the hot corn on the buttered platter and roll the ears in the dressing.

A foolproof method for tender corn:

Put the corn in enough cold water to cover. *Do not add salt.* Add the slightest pinch of sugar. If you like salt, add it just when the water comes to the boiling point. Drain immediately and the corn will be tender and ready to eat. You don't have to time corn started in cold water — just cook until the water boils.

Mayonnaise Substitute No. 1
(Makes 2½ cups)

Calories per ¼ cup: 16
Fat per ¼ cup: trace

½ cup buttermilk (made from   8 ounces nonfat yogurt
  skim)   1 teaspoon dill weed
1 cup low-fat cottage cheese

Put all the ingredients in a blender and flash blend until
smooth.

Mayonnaise Substitute No. 2
(Makes 1½ cups)

Calories per ¼ cup: 24
Fat per ¼ cup: ⅕

1 cup low-fat cottage cheese   1 tablespoon lemon juice
1 egg   Dash dry mustard, paprika, salt,
2 teaspoons vegetable oil   and pepper

Process all the ingredients in a blender until smooth.

Note: Regular mayonnaise has 400 calories and 8 fats per ¼
cup.

Butter, Margarine, Mayonnaise — All 100 percent
Fat!

Fruit Salad Dressing
(Makes 1 cup)

Calories per ¼ cup: 84
Fat per ¼ cup: ⅕

¼ cup frozen orange juice con-
    centrate
½ cup plain low-fat yogurt

¼ cup raisins
1 small apple, peeled and cored

Process all the ingredients in a blender and chill.

Russian-Style Creamy Dressing
(Makes 1½ cups)

Calories per ¼ cup: 24
Fat per ¼ cup: trace

1 8-ounce can whole tomatoes
    and liquid
½ cup low-fat cottage cheese

¼ cup pickle relish
2 tablespoons wine vinegar
1 teaspoon mustard

Combine all the ingredients in a blender.

French Dressing
(Makes 1 cup)

Calories per ¼ cup: 10
Fat per ¼ cup: trace

1 cup tomato juice
1 tablespoon white vinegar
1 teaspoon onion flakes
⅛ teaspoon basil

⅛ teaspoon dry mustard
⅛ teaspoon garlic powder
⅛ teaspoon pepper

Combine all the ingredients and chill.

Yogurt Dressing
(Makes 1 cup)

Calories per ¼ cup: 40
Fat per ¼ cup: ⅕

1 cup plain low-fat yogurt
½ teaspoon mustard
½ teaspoon salt
½ teaspoon horseradish
½ teaspoon paprika

1 clove garlic, minced
2 tablespoons lemon juice or
vinegar
1 tablespoon minced onion

Mix all the ingredients together and refrigerate.

All-Purpose Salad Dressing
(Makes 1 cup)

Calories per ¼ cup: 40
Fat per ¼ cup: ⅕

1 cup plain low-fat yogurt
½ teaspoon dill weed
⅛ teaspoon garlic powder
½ teaspoon caraway seeds
1 tablespoon wine vinegar

1 teaspoon dehydrated onion
flakes
½ packet Equal or other sugar
substitute

Mix all the ingredients and chill.

Note: Commercial salad dressings have 300 to 400 calories and
6 to 8 fats per ¼ cup.

Dressing for Cole Slaw
(Serves 5 to 6)

Calories per serving: 28
Fat per serving: trace

⅓ cup plain low-fat yogurt
1 tablespoon skim milk
1 teaspoon horseradish
1 teaspoon garlic powder

½ teaspoon salt
½ teaspoon pepper
½ medium head cabbage
1 medium carrot

Mix the first six ingredients well, pour over the grated cabbage and carrot, and toss.

Beef, Pork, and Veal

Red meat! *Red meat? Hey, what's* red meat *doing in a low-fat cookbook? Well, give heed. All red meats are not the same. Some are reasonably low in fat, especially if prepared carefully. And meat is very high in nutrition, notably protein, iron, and niacin. Meat contributes so much flavor and nutrition to recipes that we believe it's a mistake to leave it out of our diets. The trick is to buy it right, prepare it right, and, most of all, use it sparingly. Let's use meat* in *recipes rather than relying on great chunks of it as the main ingredient of a meal.*

"Un-corned beef and cabbage" . . .

Savory Beef and Cabbage
(Serves 6)

Calories per serving: 180
Fats per serving: 1½

1 pound extra-lean ground beef
1 medium onion, diced
¼ teaspoon garlic powder
½ head cabbage (about 3 cups
  coarsely shredded)
5 carrots, thinly sliced

1 bouillon cube
½ cup water
½ teaspoon salt
¼ teaspoon pepper
½ teaspoon caraway seeds

Combine the beef, onion, and garlic powder in a 2-quart casserole. Bake, uncovered, at 450° for 15 minutes, stirring occasionally to break up the meat mixture. Drain off any fat. Turn the oven to 350°. Add the cabbage and remaining ingredients; toss well. Cover the casserole and bake for 1 hour.

Browning ground beef in a skillet? You can remove
a greater amount of excess fat by placing a spoon
under one edge of the pan and cooking the meat in
the elevated portion.

Moist Meat Loaf
(Serves 8)

Calories per serving: 156
Fats per serving: 1½

3 slices whole-wheat bread
½ cup skim milk
1 pound lean ground beef
1 egg
½ cup chopped onion
1 tablespoon mustard

1 tablespoon Worcestershire
  sauce
½ teaspoon salt
½ teaspoon pepper
Ketchup

Break the bread into small pieces and soak them in the milk for
5 minutes. Add the remainder of the ingredients and mix well.
Shape into a loaf, pour a small amount of ketchup over it, and
bake at 350° for 1¼ hours.

German Bavarian Casserole
(Serves 6)

Calories per serving: 222
Fats per serving: 1½

1 14-ounce can sauerkraut and
  juice
¾ cup water
½ cup uncooked brown rice
1 medium onion, chopped

1 pound extra-lean ground beef
½ teaspoon salt
¼ teaspoon pepper
1 8-ounce can tomato sauce

Pour the sauerkraut into a 1-quart casserole and add the water. Sprinkle with the rice, then the onion, beef, salt, and pepper. Pour the tomato sauce over the top of the mixture. Bake, uncovered, at 350° for 1½ hours.

In most casseroles you can reduce the quantity of meat required by half and still get the flavor.

Ranch Stew
(Serves 4)

Calories per serving: 371
Fats per serving: 1½

1 pound lean beef, top round, trimmed and cut into bite-sized pieces	12 small canned pearl onions
	1 cup frozen peas
3 cups water	2 tablespoons whole-wheat flour (optional)
2 large carrots, pared and sliced	1 tablespoon Worcestershire sauce
2 medium potatoes, pared and diced	½ teaspoon salt
	¼ teaspoon pepper

Place the meat in a 1-quart baking dish. Brown in a slow oven at 325° for 45 minutes, stirring occasionally. Add 1 cup of water to the dish. Cover, bake for 1 hour or until the meat is tender. Meanwhile, cook the carrots in the remaining 2 cups of water in a large saucepan. When they are partially cooked, add the potatoes and cook until all the vegetables are tender. Add the onions and peas. Put the vegetables into the beef dish. Thicken the liquid from the vegetables with the flour if desired. Add the Worcestershire sauce, salt, and pepper to the liquid. Pour over the meat and vegetables. Cover, return to the oven, and cook for 20 minutes longer.

Rice Meatballs
(Serves 4)

Calories per serving: 275
Fats per serving: 2½

1 pound lean ground round
½ cup cooked brown rice
½ cup chopped green pepper
½ cup chopped onion
1 egg

½ teaspoon salt
½ teaspoon pepper
1 6-ounce can tomato paste
¾ cup water

Combine the beef, rice, green pepper, onion, egg, salt, and pepper. Mix to blend. Shape into eight meatballs. Place in a 13-by-9-by-2-inch baking dish. Bake at 375° for 30 minutes. Drain off the excess fat. Combine the tomato paste and water. Pour over the meatballs and bake for another 45 minutes.

Swiss Steak Lucerne
(Serves 4)

Calories per serving: 384
Fats per serving: 1⅕

1 pound round steak, cut about
   1 inch thick
½ teaspoon salt
Pepper
2 tablespoons whole-wheat flour

3 medium tomatoes, chopped
1 green pepper, sliced
½ cup chopped onion
4 potatoes, cubed
4 carrots, sliced

Trim the fat from the meat. Cut into serving-sized pieces. Sprinkle with half the salt, pepper, and flour. Pound the steak. Turn over and sprinkle with the rest of the salt, pepper, and flour. Pound. Place in a 9-by-11-inch oven pan. Cover with the tomatoes, pepper, and onions. Cover and bake at 325° for 2 hours. Add the potatoes and carrots and bake for 1 hour more.

Baked Beef Minestrone
(Serves 8)

This is a delicious hearty meal, but be careful if you have to watch your fats!

Calories per serving: 335
Fats per serving: 2⅕

2 pounds lean, well-trimmed
  beef stew meat
1 large onion, sliced
2 cloves garlic, minced
1 tablespoon olive oil
1 cup water
1 cup sliced carrots
1 cup sliced zucchini
1 cup diced celery
1 small green pepper
3 medium tomatoes, peeled and
  quartered

½ teaspoon salt
½ teaspoon sugar
½ teaspoon rosemary
½ teaspoon basil
½ teaspoon thyme
¼ teaspoon pepper
3 cans onion soup
3 cups shell macaroni, cooked
  and cooled
Freshly grated Parmesan
  cheese

Place the meat, onion, and garlic in the oil in a heavy kettle and bake at 400° for 40 minutes. Stir occasionally until the meat is browned. Add the water, cover, reduce the heat to 350°, and cook for 4 hours. Add the vegetables, spices, and soup, and bake for 1½ hours or until the meat is tender. To serve, spoon the macaroni into bowls and ladle the soup over it. Sprinkle with Parmesan cheese.

Country Pork Stew
(Serves 6)

Calories per serving: 260
Fats per serving: 1½

1 pound lean pork, cut into
   1-inch pieces
4 medium potatoes, unpeeled,
   cut into 1½-inch pieces
6 medium carrots, cut into
   ½-inch pieces
1 medium green pepper, cut
   into thin strips

1 medium onion, sliced
1 medium tomato, cut into thin
   wedges
2 beef bouillon cubes or envelopes
1 cup water
1 tablespoon all-purpose flour

Trim the excess fat from the pork pieces. Combine all the ingredients except the flour in a 3-quart casserole; sprinkle the
top of the mixture evenly with flour. Cover the casserole and
bake at 350°, stirring occasionally, for 2 hours or until the pork
and vegetables are tender.

For a fat-free sauce:

To remove fat from the surface of a sauce, put the
pan half on and half off the source of heat. The fat
will drift to the cooler side and can be lifted off with a
shallow-bowled spoon.

Roasting to remove fat:

If you do not have a roasting rack and want to keep
the underside of the meat from frying in its own fat,
use two or three metal jar lids with holes punched in
the tops. The roast will sit on top of the punched lids
and the hot dry air in the oven will be able to circu-
late freely.

Macaroni Carbonara
(Serves 4)

We found this tasty recipe in The Joy of Cooking. *The original calls for ½ pound of ham, 2 tablespoons of butter, and 1 teaspoon of salt, for a total of 541 calories and 2 fats per serving.*

Calories per serving: 285
Fat per serving: 1

2 cups dry elbow macaroni
3 quarts boiling water
½ teaspoon salt
¼ pound ham, in chunks
¼ cup parsley sprigs

2 stalks celery, chopped
1 small onion, quartered
1 small green pepper, chopped
1 egg
Dash pepper

Cook the macaroni in the water and salt until tender. Drain. Finely chop the ham, parsley, celery, onion, and green pepper. Sauté in 2 tablespoons water in a large skillet until tender. Mix in the macaroni. Beat together the egg and pepper. Mix into the macaroni until blended and heat through.

Select Lean Cuts of Beef!

3½ ounces of the following cooked meats, trimmed of fat and untrimmed, yield dramatically different amounts of fat.

	Trimmed No. of Fats	Untrimmed No. of Fats
Round steak	1	2³/₅
Leg of lamb	1⅕	3⅕
Flank steak	1⅕	3
Rump roast	1³/₅	4³/₅
Sirloin steak	1³/₅	5³/₅
Ground beef, lean with 10% fat	2	—
Boneless chuck	2²/₅	6⅕

Veal and Lima Beans
(Serves 4)

Calories per serving: 340
Fat per serving: 1

2 pounds fresh lima beans
¼ cup lemon juice
1 medium onion, diced
½ pound veal, sliced
¼ cup red wine

1 tablespoon chopped parsley
½ teaspoon dill weed
¾ cup tomato purée
¼ cup water

Shell the beans. Cover with boiling water. Add the lemon juice and cook uncovered for about 30 minutes or until tender. Drain. While the beans are cooking, brown the onion in a nonstick pan until golden. Remove from the pan. Brown the veal in the same pan. Place all the ingredients in a casserole and mix together. Bake, uncovered, at 350° for 1 hour.

Poultry

Chicken Paprika
(Serves 5)

Calories per serving: 320
Fats per serving: 1³/₅

2 teaspoons vegetable oil
1 cup coarsely chopped onion
¼ teaspoon garlic powder
4 teaspoons paprika
¼ teaspoon pepper
1 cup chicken bouillon
2 tablespoons cornstarch

½ cup water
2 cups skinned and cooked
 chicken or turkey
1 cup frozen peas
1 cup plain low-fat yogurt
2 cups hot cooked noodles

Heat the oil in a large skillet and add the onion, garlic powder, paprika, and pepper. Cook until tender, stirring frequently. Add the bouillon. Blend the cornstarch in the water and add to the skillet; stir until smooth. Bring to a boil, stirring constantly, and add the chicken and peas. Boil for 1 minute. Remove from the heat; stir in the yogurt until blended. Serve over the noodles.

When you skin a chicken *before* cooking, you remove about 55 percent of the calories. When you skin it *after* cooking, some of the fat has soaked into the meat and you remove only about 25 percent of the calories.

Chicken Napoli
(Serves 6)

Calories per serving: 240
Fat per serving: ⁴⁄₅

1 fryer, skinned and cut into
  serving pieces
½ cauliflower, separated into
  florets
2 potatoes, pared and diced
2 carrots, pared and sliced
½ eggplant, unpared and cubed
2 onions, sliced
1 red or green pepper, sliced

2 stalks celery, cut in diagonal
  slices
½ teaspoon pepper
1 16-ounce can tomatoes
½ teaspoon garlic powder
2 teaspoons chicken bouillon
  powder
1½ cups water
1 tablespoon dill weed

Place the chicken and vegetables in a 4-quart casserole. Sprinkle with pepper. Add the tomatoes, garlic powder, bouillon powder, and water. Sprinkle with dill. Cover tightly and bake at 350° for 2 hours. Stir after 1 hour. The flavor continues to develop as the casserole stands.

Chicken Risotto
(Serves 8)

Calories per serving: 187
Fat per serving: 1

2 small zucchini, thinly sliced
2 green onions, sliced
2 cups skinned and cooked
  diced chicken
½ teaspoon salt

½ teaspoon thyme
2 tablespoons chopped pimiento
3 cups cooked whole-grain rice
¼ cup grated cheese*

* When you use a strong aged cheese, you can cut down on the quantity and still retain the flavor.

Cook the zucchini and onions in a small amount of water until tender — about 5 to 10 minutes. Add the other ingredients, except for the cheese. Cook and stir until heated through. Remove from the heat, stir in the cheese, and serve.

Chicken and Fresh Vegetables Provençale
(Serves 4)

Calories per serving: 220
Fat per serving: ³⁄₅

1 small head cauliflower
2 large ripe tomatoes, sliced
2 medium carrots, pared and thinly sliced
1 large onion, thinly sliced
2 tablespoons chopped fresh parsley, divided
1 tablespoon diced leaf basil, divided

¼ teaspoon pepper
1 chicken bouillon cube
½ cup boiling water
1 teaspoon garlic powder
2 tablespoons lemon juice
2 whole chicken breasts, skinned and split

Break the cauliflower into small pieces. Combine the vegetables in a 3-quart baking dish. Sprinkle with 1 tablespoon parsley, 2 teaspoons basil, and the pepper. Combine the bouillon cube and the water and pour over the vegetables. Make a paste of 1 tablespoon parsley, 1 teaspoon basil, the garlic powder, and the lemon juice. Place the chicken over the vegetables. Spread the paste on the chicken. Cover and bake at 350° for 1½ hours or until the chicken and vegetables are tender, basting occasionally.

East Indian Chicken
(Serves 4)

Calories per serving: 340
Fats per serving: 1⅖

½ cup chopped onion
½ cup chopped green pepper
¼ teaspoon garlic powder
1 teaspoon vegetable oil
2 cups skinned and cooked
   diced chicken
½ teaspoon salt
½ teaspoon pepper

1½ teaspoons curry powder
1 28-ounce can whole tomatoes
1 tablespoon Worcestershire
   sauce
2 tablespoons chopped parsley
¼ cup raisins (optional)
2 cups cooked brown rice

Cook the onion, pepper, and garlic powder in the oil until the onion is tender — about 3 minutes. Add the remaining ingredients, except the rice, and cook over low heat for about 30 minutes. Serve over the rice.

Chicken, Bean, and Rice Casserole
(Serves 6)

Calories per serving: 220
Fat per serving: ⅗

3 cups cooked brown rice
1 tablespoon chopped fresh
   parsley
1 cup chicken broth
½ cup skim milk
3 tablespoons flour
¼ teaspoon salt

¼ teaspoon pepper
1½ cups skinned and cooked
   cubed chicken
1 pound fresh or canned green
   beans cooked with 1 tablespoon onion flakes
½ cup sliced fresh mushrooms

Combine the rice and parsley in an 8-by-12-inch nonstick baking dish. Make a white sauce of the broth, milk, flour, salt, and pepper. Combine the chicken, beans, mushrooms, and sauce, and place the mixture over the rice. Cover and bake at 350° for 35 to 40 minutes. If desired, sprinkle fresh chopped onion over the top and bake uncovered for 5 minutes longer.

Chicken or Turkey Strata
(Serves 8)

Although this recipe has been modified from one with a much higher fat content, 3 fats may still be too high for some of you. But, oh, it's good!

Calories per serving: 328
Fats per serving: 3

8 slices whole-wheat bread, cut into 1-inch cubes
2 cups skinned and cooked cubed turkey or chicken
½ cup finely chopped onion
⅔ cup finely chopped celery
1 4-ounce can diced green chilies (optional)
½ cup reduced-fat mayonnaise (Light 'n Lively)

½ teaspoon salt
¼ teaspoon pepper
3 corn tortillas
3 eggs, slightly beaten
1¾ cups 2% low-fat milk
1 cup low-fat cottage cheese
1 10¾-ounce can condensed cream of mushroom soup

Place the cubes of bread on the bottom of a 12-by-18-inch nonstick pan. Combine the chicken, onion, celery, chilies, mayonnaise, salt, and pepper in a medium-sized bowl, and spoon over the bread cubes. Tear the tortillas into bite-sized pieces and place them on top of the chicken mixture. Combine the eggs, milk, cottage cheese, and soup in a small bowl and pour over the top. Cover and refrigerate overnight to allow the flavors to blend. Preheat the oven to 325° and bake for 50 minutes to 1 hour or until the dish is firm and set. Remove from the oven and let stand for 10 minutes before serving.

Chicken and Sweet Potato Bake
(Serves 6)

Calories per serving: 280
Fat per serving: 4/5

3 medium sweet potatoes,
  peeled and cut into small
  chunks
3 whole chicken breasts,
  skinned and split
1 small onion, diced

1 celery stalk, diced
½ cup apple juice
2 teaspoons chicken bouillon
  powder
2 9-ounce packages frozen cut
  green beans, thawed

Put all the ingredients in a 3-quart casserole; toss well. Cover and bake, stirring occasionally, at 375° for 1 hour or until the chicken is tender.

Chicken Livers in Wine
(Serves 4)

We didn't believe how good this dish could be until we tried it in our kitchens. Give yourself a treat and forget "how it sounds."

Calories per serving: 159
Fat per serving: 4/5

1 large onion, chopped
2 tablespoons water
½ pound fresh mushrooms,
  sliced
½ pound chicken livers, cut in
  halves

1 tablespoon flour
1 tablespoon butter
½ cup red wine
1 cup plain low-fat yogurt
1 teaspoon soy sauce
Pepper to taste

Sauté the onion in the water until soft. Add the mushrooms and sauté for 3 to 4 minutes. Dust the livers with the flour and sauté them in the butter in a separate pan until they lose their pink color. Combine the wine, yogurt, and soy sauce. Combine the mushrooms and livers and pour the sauce over them. Season with pepper and cook the mixture over low heat until the livers are done.

Chicken, Beans, and Vegetables
(Serves 8 to 10)

Covert likes to add a couple of tablespoons of low-fat cottage cheese to this dish for a completely balanced four-food-group meal.

Calories per serving: 275
Fat per serving: $2/5$

5 whole chicken breasts, skinned and split	½ teaspoon basil
	½ teaspoon thyme
4 quarts water	Pepper
½ cup dry lima beans, washed	1 teaspoon salt
1 cup dry pinto beans, washed	3 to 4 carrots, sliced
2 onions, chopped	3 to 4 stalks celery, sliced
½ cup pearl barley	1 cup frozen peas
2 to 3 tomatoes, cut up	

Combine the chicken, water, and lima beans in a large pot. Bring to a boil, cover, and simmer for 30 minutes. Add the pinto beans and onion. Simmer for 1 hour. Remove the chicken. Add the barley, tomatoes, and seasonings. Simmer for another hour. Add the carrots and celery. Cook over medium-low heat until the carrots are tender. Remove the chicken from the bones and cut it into small pieces. Add the chicken and peas to the pot. Cook until the peas are tender — about 5 minutes.

Chicken and Rice
(Serves 4)

Sure, you've eaten this before. Probably with a multitude of fats.
Now delight in a new flavor with less than a single fat.

Calories per serving: 300
Fat per serving: $3/5$

1 cup skinned and cooked
   cubed chicken
2 cups cooked brown rice
2 raw zucchini, unpeeled and
   cut into bite-sized pieces
2 cups frozen chopped spinach,
   defrosted and drained

½ teaspoon tarragon
½ teaspoon pepper
½ teaspoon paprika
½ teaspoon onion powder
1 cup sherry

Mix all the ingredients, except the sherry, together and pour
into a baking dish. Pour the sherry over the entire mixture.
Cover and bake at 350° for 40 minutes.

Orange Baked Chicken
(Serves 6)

Calories per serving: 220
Fat per serving: $4/5$

3 whole chicken breasts,
   skinned and split
¼ cup minced onion
½ teaspoon paprika
½ teaspoon salt

¼ teaspoon rosemary
¼ teaspoon pepper
2 tablespoons flour
2 cups orange juice

Arrange the chicken in a shallow baking pan, breast side up,
not overlapping. Sprinkle with the onion and seasonings.

Blend the flour with ½ cup orange juice; stir in the remaining juice and pour over the chicken. Bake, uncovered, basting occasionally, at 350° for 1 hour or until tender. Serve the chicken over noodles or rice on a warm platter. Stir the pan juices to blend and pour over the chicken.

Chicken Curry
(Serves 6)

You don't like turnips — or always thought you didn't? Try this tasty mind changer. You won't even realize you're eating turnips!

Calories per serving: 285
Fat per serving: ⅘

3 whole chicken breasts, skinned and split
1 16-ounce can tomatoes
1 medium onion, diced
⅛ teaspoon garlic powder
1½ cups boiling water
6 medium turnips, peeled and diced

¾ cup brown rice
1 tablespoon curry powder
2 teaspoons sugar
¾ teaspoon salt
¼ teaspoon ground ginger
⅛ teaspoon pepper

Arrange the chicken in a 2½-quart casserole. Bake, uncovered, at 450° for about 10 to 15 minutes. Turn the temperature to 375°. Add the tomatoes and stir to break them up. Add the remaining ingredients and stir well. Cover and bake for 1 hour or until the rice is cooked and the turnips are tender. Stir occasionally.

Hot Chicken Salad
(Serves 6)

Calories per serving: 140
Fat per serving: ⁴/₅

2 cups skinned and cooked
  bite-sized pieces chicken
½ cup plain low-fat yogurt
2 teaspoons grated onion
½ teaspoon curry

1 cup chopped celery
1 8½-ounce can water chestnuts, cut
½ pound fresh mushrooms,
  sliced

Mix all the ingredients together and pour into an 8½-inch-square casserole. Bake, uncovered, at 450° for 10 minutes. Serve hot.

Carla's Turkey Loaf*
(Serves 8)

Ground turkey is an excellent substitute for ground beef, cutting the fat content by more than a third. It can be used for any casserole in which you would ordinarily use ground beef and also in tacos, spaghetti, lasagna, or burgers. Its bland flavor assumes the seasonings of the dish and therefore serves as a good masquerade for your meat-loving guests.

Calories per serving: 184
Fats per serving: 1³/₅

2 pounds ground turkey
2 tablespoons hot ketchup
1 tablespoon Worcestershire
  sauce
1 medium onion, chopped
1 teaspoon salt
½ teaspoon pepper

1 stalk celery, finely chopped
1 teaspoon rosemary
1 teaspoon thyme
1 teaspoon basil
2 tablespoons chopped parsley
½ cup oatmeal

* From *Lean Life Cuisine* by Carla Mulligan and Eve Lowry

Mix all the ingredients together and form into a loaf. Place in a nonstick loaf pan and bake at 350° for 2 hours.

Turkey Sausages
(Serves 8)

These sausages can be preshaped, wrapped individually, and frozen until needed.

Calories per sausage: 95
Fat per sausage: ½

1 pound ground turkey	½ teaspoon pepper
1 teaspoon salt	1 teaspoon sage

Combine all the ingredients and mix well. Refrigerate for a few hours or overnight to let the flavors mingle and develop. Shape into 8 patties. Cook, but do not overcook, over medium heat. High cooking temperatures make for a tough sausage, and overcooking can result in a very dry one. Remember, there's not much fat in ground turkey.

Variations
For milder, low-salt sausages:
Mix 1 pound ground turkey with ½ teaspoon thyme, ⅛ teaspoon nutmeg, and ¼ teaspoon ginger.

Mix 1 pound ground turkey with 2 minced garlic cloves, ½ teaspoon thyme, and ¼ teaspoon rosemary.

Mix 1 pound ground turkey with 2 minced garlic cloves, ¼ teaspoon oregano, and ¼ teaspoon basil.

For spicier sausages:
Add to the basic recipe ½ teaspoon thyme, ¼ teaspoon cayenne pepper, and ½ teaspoon coriander.

> **Pork Sausage:**
>
> Calories per sausage: 112
> Fats per sausage: 1 ½

Fish and Seafood

Fish Florentine Casserole
(Serves 4 to 5)

Calories per serving: 233
Fat per serving: ½

1 pound frozen fish fillets
1 small onion, minced
1 teaspoon margarine
1½ cups skim milk
1½ teaspoons chicken bouillon
  powder
¼ teaspoon paprika

1½ tablespoons cornstarch
4 medium potatoes, peeled and
  thinly sliced
1 10-ounce package frozen
  chopped spinach, thawed and
  squeezed dry

Thaw the fish fillets slightly at room temperature for 15 to 30 minutes. Cook the onion in margarine until tender. Stir in 1 cup of the milk, the bouillon, and the paprika. Mix the cornstarch with the remaining ½ cup milk, then add to the milk and onion mixture. Stir constantly over medium heat until the mixture thickens. Cut the fillets into ¼-inch slices with a sharp knife. Arrange half the potatoes in a layer in a 2½-quart casserole, top with half the spinach, then half the fish, then half the sauce. Repeat. Cover the casserole and bake at 375° for 1½ hours or until the potatoes are tender.

Poached Salmon Steaks
with Cucumber Sauce
(Serves 4)

We love salmon, but it is higher in fat than most other fish. If you are eating from Category 2 or 3 (see the table at the beginning of this book), use sole instead.

Calories per salmon serving: 250
Fats per salmon serving: 2½

Calories per sole serving: 96
Fat per sole serving: ⅕

2 cups boiling water
2 chicken bouillon cubes
1 tablespoon vinegar
1 small onion, sliced
1 teaspoon dill weed

⅛ teaspoon salt
¼ teaspoon pepper
2 salmon steaks, about 1 inch
  thick

Combine all the ingredients, except the salmon, in a skillet over high heat. Reduce the heat to low. Cover and simmer for 5 minutes. Add the salmon. Cover and simmer for 8 minutes or until the fish flakes easily. Remove the bones and cut each steak in half. Place the drained onion slices over the steaks and top with Cucumber Sauce. Serve at room temperature.

Cucumber Sauce

½ cup finely diced cucumber,
  drained
¼ cup Mock Sour Cream No. 2
  (see Sauces, Dips, and Dressings)

¼ teaspoon celery salt
¼ teaspoon pepper

Mix all the ingredients together.

Fish Creole
(Serves 6)

Nice mild creole.

Calories per serving: 165
Fat per serving: ¹/₁₀

1 16-ounce package frozen cod or other fillets
1 16-ounce can tomatoes
1 medium onion, diced
1 medium green pepper, diced
¼ teaspoon garlic powder
¾ cup uncooked regular long-grain rice

½ cup water
2 tablespoons minced parsley
½ teaspoon salt
½ teaspoon paprika
¼ teaspoon hot pepper sauce

Thaw the fish fillets slightly and cut them into bite-sized pieces. Combine all the ingredients in a 2-quart casserole, and stir to break up the tomatoes. Cover and bake at 375° for 1¼ hours or until the fish and rice are tender. Stir once after 45 minutes.

Baked Flounder
(Serves 4)

Calories per serving: 130
Fat per serving: ¹/₅

1 cup tomato juice
½ cup sliced fresh mushrooms
1 teaspoon lemon juice

1 small onion, cut in quarters
Salt and pepper to taste
1½ pounds flounder

Place all the ingredients, except the fish, in a pan and bring to a boil. Lower the heat and cook for 5 minutes. Wipe the fish clean with a damp cloth, place it in a shallow baking dish, and pour the sauce over it. Bake at 375°, basting several times, for 25 minutes.

Seafood Stroganoff
(Serves 4)

Calories per serving: 248
Fat per serving: $2/5$

Juice of 1 lemon
1 ½ pounds white fish
1 medium onion, chopped
1 cup sherry
½ pound fresh mushrooms,
   sliced

1 cup Mock Sour Cream No. 2
   (see Sauces, Dips, and Dressings)
½ teaspoon basil
1 tablespoon chopped fresh
   parsley

Pour the lemon juice on both sides of the fish. Sauté the onion in ½ cup of the sherry until golden brown. Add the mushrooms and sauté until tender. Spray a broiler pan with nonstick spray. Place the fish on the pan under the broiler. Broil, turning once, until golden brown on each side. While the fish is broiling, add the remaining sherry and the Mock Sour Cream, basil, and parsley to the onion and mushroom mixture. Simmer over low heat until just heated through. Pour over the fish. Serve immediately.

Skillet Fish with Vegetables
(Serves 4)

Calories per serving: 110
Fat per serving: $1/10$

4 tablespoons finely chopped
   onion
¼ teaspoon garlic powder
1 cup finely chopped carrots
1 cup thinly sliced mushrooms
1 cup coarsely chopped tomatoes

2 tablespoons chopped parsley
½ teaspoon basil leaves
¼ teaspoon pepper
½ teaspoon salt
1 pound fish fillets (flounder,
   haddock, or sole)
2 tablespoons lemon juice

Simmer all the ingredients, except the fish and lemon juice, for about 20 minutes or until the carrots are tender. Add the fish and lemon juice, spooning the vegetables over the fish. Cover and cook for 15 minutes longer or until the fish flakes easily.

Creamy Salmon Casserole
(Serves 6)

Beware! Salmon is a fatty fish.

Calories per serving: 277
Fats per serving: 3

1 15½-ounce can salmon	¼ teaspoon salt
1 teaspoon margarine	½ teaspoon dill weed
1 medium celery stalk, diced	1 10-ounce package frozen
1 medium green pepper, diced	peas, thawed
1 cup skim milk	4 hard-boiled eggs, sliced
1½ tablespoons cornstarch, softened in 1½ tablespoons cold water	

Drain the salmon, reserving the liquid, and flake it. Melt the margarine in a saucepan, add the celery and green pepper, and cook until tender — about 5 minutes. Stir in the milk and salmon liquid. When hot, add the cornstarch and water, stirring constantly until thick. Season with the salt and dill weed. Arrange half the peas in a 1½-quart casserole, then half the egg slices, then half the salmon. Repeat. Gradually spoon the sauce on the top. Cover and bake at 375° for 25 minutes or until heated through.

Examine fish to be sure it is fresh. It must be firm and have tight scales and a bright color. The eyes should be clear, moist, and bulging. If the fish smells particularly strong, it is not fresh.

Peppery Tuna Casserole
(Serves 8)

Calories per serving: 118
Fat per serving: ⅕

8 ounces macaroni
1 ½ cups skim milk
3 tablespoons cornstarch
½ cup water
1 4-ounce can mushroom
  pieces, drained

½ teaspoon thyme
¼ teaspoon pepper
2 medium zucchini, sliced
1 6½-ounce can water-packed
  tuna, drained
½ cup sliced radishes

Cook the macaroni as directed. Drain. Put the milk in a small saucepan and heat. Soften the cornstarch in the water and slowly add to the milk, stirring constantly, to make a thick sauce. Add the mushrooms, thyme, and pepper. Arrange half the macaroni in a 2½-quart deep casserole; top with half the zucchini, then half the tuna, then half the radishes. Repeat. Spoon the sauce mixture over the top layer. Cover the casserole and bake at 375° for about 45 minutes or until it is heated through and the zucchini is tender.

Tuna Salad
(Serves 4)

Calories per serving: 170
Fat per serving: ⅖

1 medium tomato, chopped fine
2 pimientos, chopped fine
½ cup chopped celery
3 green onions, chopped fine
2 dill pickles, chopped fine
1 6½-ounce can water-packed
  tuna, flaked

½ cucumber, chopped fine
Salt and pepper to taste
¾ cup Mayonnaise Substitute
  No. 1 (see Sauces, Dips, and
  Dressings)

Mix all the ingredients together and refrigerate.

Herb Crab (or Creole, If You Prefer)
(Serves 2)

Calories per serving: 115
Fat per serving: ½

2 cleaned, cooked fresh crabs
  (or 1 large can crabmeat if
  fresh unavailable)
½ cup water or wine
2 teaspoons garlic powder
1 teaspoon onion powder

1 teaspoon basil
1 teaspoon paprika
½ fresh green pepper, chopped
½ fresh onion, thinly sliced,
  chopped

Crack the crab legs slightly. Sauté all the ingredients in the water or wine (no oil). Simmer together for 1 hour, adding liquid if necessary, or microwave for 10 to 12 minutes, stirring twice.

For creole style, substitute 1 can tomato sauce for the liquid and add 2 to 3 drops (or more, to suit your taste) of Tabasco sauce.

Shrimp Casserole
(Serves 4)

Calories per serving: 158
Fat per serving: ⅕

1 cup cooked brown rice
1 pound shrimp, peeled and
  deveined
½ cup minced onion
1 bay leaf

3 cups peeled and chopped
  tomatoes
1 teaspoon chili powder
½ teaspoon salt
½ teaspoon pepper

Toss all the ingredients together and bake in a covered casserole at 350° for 30 minutes.

Stuffed Pitas
(Serves 6)

Calories per serving: 249
Fat per serving: $\frac{2}{5}$

1 cup bulgar wheat
1 cucumber, chopped
2 tomatoes, chopped
1 teaspoon Dijon mustard
2 teaspoons red wine vinegar
⅓ cup lemon juice

1 pound cooked shrimp, peeled
and deveined (or crab, water-
packed tuna, skinned chicken
or turkey)
6 whole-wheat pita bread
pockets
6 leaves of lettuce

Prepare the bulgar according to the directions on the package, soaking in water for 1 hour. Combine the bulgar with the other ingredients in a large mixing bowl. Cut the meat into bite-sized pieces if necessary. Split open the pitas, insert a lettuce leaf in each, and stuff them with the salad mixture.

Beans and
Other Legumes

Lentil Burgers with Dill Sauce
(Makes 8)

Calories per burger, bun, and sauce: 240
Fat per burger, bun, and sauce: $2/5$

1 cup lentils
3 cups water
½ cup diced onion
½ teaspoon salt
¼ teaspoon pepper
2 slices crumbled whole-wheat bread
2 tablespoons whole-wheat flour
2 egg whites

1 tablespoon horseradish
1 teaspoon Worcestershire sauce
1 tablespoon Dijon mustard
½ teaspoon oregano
¼ teaspoon thyme
¼ teaspoon sage
¼ teaspoon basil

Cook the first five ingredients together until all the water is absorbed — about 40 minutes. Then add the remaining ingredients and mix well. Divide into eight portions, spoon onto a nonstick surface, and flatten to the size of burger desired. Cook on both sides until light brown. Serve with Dill Sauce on whole-wheat buns.

Dill Sauce

½ cup buttermilk (made from skim)
1 cup low-fat cottage cheese

1 cup nonfat yogurt
1 teaspoon dill weed

Combine all the ingredients in a blender and process until smooth. Spoon over the burgers.

Lentil Curry Stew
(Serves 6)

Calories per serving: 334
Fat per serving: $\frac{1}{5}$

2 cups dried lentils
½ cup chopped onion
2 to 3 cloves garlic, minced
¼ cup chicken bouillon
½ teaspoon curry powder

3 cups water
5 potatoes, cut up
1 tomato, cut up
2 cups skim milk
Juice of ½ lemon

Wash the lentils. Sauté the onion and garlic in the bouillon until the onions are slightly golden. Add the curry powder, water, and lentils. Bring to a boil. Reduce the heat and simmer for 15 to 20 minutes. Add the potatoes, tomato, and milk. Cover and continue cooking until the potatoes are tender when pierced. Remove from the heat. Add the lemon juice and serve.

Lima Bean Loaf
(Serves 6)

Without peanuts:
Calories per serving: 283
Fats per serving: 1 ½

With peanuts:
Calories per serving: 374
Fats per serving: 2 ½

1 cup dry lima beans
2 tablespoons margarine
1 small onion, chopped
1 cup thinly sliced celery
¼ cup whole-wheat flour
1 cup skim milk
1 egg, beaten
1 cup soft, fine whole-wheat
   bread crumbs

1 ½ cups chopped or grated
   carrots
¾ teaspoon salt
¼ teaspoon pepper
½ cup chopped peanuts
   (optional)

Soak the beans overnight in cold water. Drain, rinse, and cook in water to cover until tender — about 1½ hours. Drain the beans and mash them. Melt the margarine in a saucepan. Add the onion and sauté for about 3 minutes. Add the celery, cover, and cook until tender. Add the flour and cook for 2 minutes. Add the milk, stirring until thickened. Remove from the heat and stir in the egg. Add the crumbs, carrots, salt, pepper, and peanuts. Spoon the mixture into an 8-by-4-inch nonstick loaf pan and bake at 375° for 35 to 45 minutes.

When you sauté:

Use one-third the amount of fat usually suggested. Better yet, use water or bouillon and nonstick cookware.

Corn and Bean Main Dish
(Serves 10)

Calories per serving: 302
Fats per serving: 1⅕

4 cups cooked pinto beans	¼ cup margarine
2 cups dry cornmeal	1 quart buttermilk (made from
2 teaspoons baking soda	skim)
1 teaspoon salt	3 egg whites, slightly beaten

Spread the beans over the bottom of an 8-by-12-inch casserole. Mix the dry ingredients in a large bowl. Melt the margarine and combine with the buttermilk and egg whites. Stir the wet and dry ingredients together until smooth and pour over the beans. The mixture will be very wet. Bake at 450° on the top rack of the oven for 30 minutes or until the bread is a golden color and its sides pull away from the pan. Cut in large squares while hot and serve.

Vegetarian Lentils
(Serves 4)

Calories per serving: 190
Fat per serving: $\frac{1}{10}$

1 onion, chopped
½ teaspoon vegetable oil
2 cloves garlic, minced
5 mushrooms, sliced
¼ cup pearl barley

1 teaspoon cumin
½ teaspoon lemon juice
Salt and pepper to taste
2 cups water
¾ cup lentils

Brown the onion in the oil until golden. Add the garlic and mushrooms and stir thoroughly. Add the barley and cumin and stir again. Add the lemon juice and salt and pepper, then the water and lentils. Cover and cook slowly for 45 minutes, adding more water if necessary.

Lenten Cabbage Rolls
(Serves 8)

Calories per serving: 270
Fat per serving: 1

1 large head cabbage
1½ cups bulgar wheat
1 8-ounce can garbanzo beans,
   drained
2 tomatoes, cut up
1 bunch parsley, chopped
1 medium onion, chopped

4 lemons
2 tablespoons vegetable oil
1 teaspoon salt
Dash pepper
1 clove garlic
1 tablespoon dried mint

Core the cabbage and place it in salted boiling water. Separate the leaves and parboil. Take the leaves from the cabbage one at a time. Cut the leaves in half and remove the vein. Wash the bulgar thoroughly, squeeze out the water, and mix it with the garbanzo beans, tomatoes, parsley, onion, juice of 3 lemons, oil, salt, and pepper. Place 1 tablespoon of the mixture in a cabbage leaf and roll. Line the bottom of a large skillet with cabbage rolls. Add the garlic, mint, and the juice of 1 lemon and cover with an inverted plate. Pour water to plate level. Remove the plate, cover the skillet, and bring to a boil. Reduce the heat and cook for 20 minutes.

French Bean Casserole
(Serves 8)

The original recipe used double the bacon, pork, and pepperoni of this one. By cutting back, we retained the flavor of these meats and eliminated 50 percent of the fat calories.

Calories per serving: 383
Fat per serving: 1⅗

2 cups dried white navy beans
4 slices bacon
1 carrot, cut into ¼-inch slices
1 medium onion, stuck with
  2 cloves
½ teaspoon garlic powder
Salt and pepper to taste
½ pound lean pork, cut into
  cubes

2 ounces pepperoni, sliced
2 large onions, chopped
1 cup diced celery
2 tablespoons tomato paste
4 beef bouillon cubes dissolved
  in 3 cups hot water
2 cups bread crumbs

Soak the beans overnight and drain. Line a large casserole with the bacon. Mix the beans, carrot, whole onion, ¼ teaspoon garlic powder, salt, and pepper. Pour into the casserole, cover with water, and bake at 275° for 2 hours. Meanwhile, put the other ingredients, except the bread crumbs, in a pot and simmer for 1½ hours, stirring occasionally. Empty the meat mixture into the casserole, stir well, and stir in the crumbs. Increase the heat to 375° and bake for about 15 minutes more.

Black Beans and Rice
(Serves 8)

Calories per serving: 275
Fat per serving: 1

1 pound black beans
1 large onion, chopped
1 clove garlic, mashed
1 green pepper, chopped
2 teaspoons olive oil
1 ham hock, small (¼ pound);
   trim fat

1 teaspoon oregano
3 bay leaves
½ cup vinegar
2 cups cooked brown rice

Wash the beans and soak overnight in 2 quarts of cold water. Sauté the onion (and it's just as good if you leave the onion raw), garlic, and pepper in the oil. Combine all the ingredients, except the vinegar and rice, and cook over low heat until the beans are tender. Add the vinegar and serve over the rice.

Lentil-Rice Tostados
(Serves 8)

Calories per serving: 250
Fat per serving: $1/10$

1 pound lentils
5 cups water
1 cup tomato sauce
1 cup chopped or stewed tomatoes
1 medium onion, chopped
2 cloves garlic, minced
¼ cup chopped green pepper

3 to 4 tablespoons chili powder
Salt to taste (optional)
2 cups cooked brown rice
Shredded lettuce
Alfalfa sprouts
Chopped tomatoes
Plain nonfat yogurt

Simmer the lentils in the water for 30 minutes. Add the tomato sauce, tomatoes, onion, garlic, green pepper, chili powder, and salt, and simmer for an additional 30 minutes, stirring frequently. Spoon the lentil mixture onto a platter of rice and layer with the remaining ingredients.

As a general rule of thumb:

- One cup of any dry legume will yield two cups of the cooked product.
- All legumes (except split peas, black-eyed peas, and lentils) require presoaking. Use either of the following methods.
  a. Cover the beans with cold water (so that the water is 1 inch above the beans) and soak overnight.
  b. Cover the beans with hot water (so that the water is 1 inch above the beans), boil for 2 minutes, and soak for at least 1 hour.

Lentils with Rice
(Serves 8)

Calories per serving: 200
Fat per serving: ½

1 cup lentils	1 small onion, diced
3½ cups water	1 large onion, cut into wedges
1 teaspoon salt	1 tablespoon oil
1 cup brown rice	

Wash the lentils, add the water and salt, and boil for 10 minutes in a covered saucepan. Wash the rice; add it and the diced onion to the lentils; stir and cover. Cook over low heat for 45 minutes longer. Sauté the onion wedges in the oil until golden brown. Place the lentils and rice on a serving platter and top with the sautéed onions.

Beans 'n' Bran
(Serves 2)

Once the beans have been cooked, this dish is very good served as a quick snack. The bran adds body to the mixture and thickens it to lend a molasseslike consistency.

Calories per serving: 200
Fat per serving: $1/5$

1 cup cooked beans (navy or
   great northern)
½ cup water
½ cup ketchup

¼ cup 100% all-bran cereal
1 teaspoon chili powder
3 dashes Tabasco sauce

Mix the ingredients in a saucepan and stir well. Boil for 2 to 3 minutes.

Spinach and Garbanzo Beans with Cheese
(Serves 6)

Calories per serving: 313
Fats per serving: $2 1/5$

3 cups cooked garbanzo beans,
   drained
½ cup bean liquid
1 tablespoon olive oil
1 pound spinach, chopped

1 teaspoon cumin
1 tablespoon lemon juice
8 ounces (about 1⅓ cups) part-
   skim mozzarella cheese
Pepper to taste

Combine the beans, liquid, oil, spinach, and cumin in a large pot; cover and cook over low heat until the spinach is tender and everything else is hot — about 5 to 10 minutes. Stir in the lemon juice, crumble in the cheese, add a generous amount of pepper, and remove from the heat. Serve hot or at room temperature.

Lentil Stew
(Serves 8)

Calories per 1½-cup serving: 250
Fat per 1½-cup serving: ⅘

2 tablespoons butter or margarine
1 cup chopped onion
1 clove garlic, minced
6 cups water
1 pound dried lentils, washed
1 teaspoon Worcestershire sauce
½ teaspoon oregano
1 bay leaf
6 large carrots, cut into ½-inch pieces
4 large stalks celery, cut into 1-inch pieces
1 teaspoon salt
1 16-ounce can tomato pieces
½ cup chopped parsley

Melt the butter in a large skillet. Sauté the onion and garlic until the onion is tender. Add the water, lentils, Worcestershire sauce, oregano, and bay leaf. Cover and bring to a boil, reduce the heat, and simmer for 45 minutes. Add the carrots, celery, and salt. Cover and simmer for 30 minutes longer or until the vegetables are tender. Add the tomatoes and heat. Remove the bay leaf. Turn into a serving dish. Garnish with parsley.

Rice and Pasta

Macaroni Loaf
(Serves 5)

This is a very attractive dish. We found the recipe in The Joy of Cooking, *where it calls for whole milk, 2 tablespoons butter, 2 eggs, and cheddar cheese. The original recipe has 233 calories and 2⅖ fats per serving.*

Calories per serving: 175
Fat per serving: ⅘

¾ cup dry macaroni
¾ teaspoon salt
5 cups water
½ cup skim milk
1 egg
2 teaspoons butter or margarine
½ cup soft bread crumbs

1 cup low-fat cottage cheese
2 tablespoons sliced pimientos
¼ cup chopped green pepper
⅛ teaspoon salt
⅛ teaspoon paprika
⅛ teaspoon pepper

Boil the macaroni in the salted water for 20 minutes or until tender. Drain in a colander and pour 2 cups cold water over it. Place in a bowl. Scald the milk and beat the egg into it. Melt the butter and add it to the milk. Pour over the macaroni. Add the remaining ingredients. Put the mixture in a nonstick baking dish and bake at 350° for 30 to 45 minutes.

Noodle Casserole
(Serves 8)

Calories per serving: 182
Fat per serving: ⅘

½ pound spinach noodles	Salt and pepper to taste
1 cup plain low-fat yogurt	½ cup raisins soaked in rum
1 cup low-fat cottage cheese	¼ cup slivered almonds

Cook the noodles; drain. Toss with the other ingredients. Put in a casserole and bake at 350° for 20 minutes or until bubbling hot. This is a good accompaniment to baked ham.

Garden Pasta
(Serves 6 to 8)

If you were in Firenze, Roma, or Napoli and ordered this dish, you'd almost trade your passport for the recipe. Enjoy it, with our compliments.

Calories per serving: 150
Fat per serving: ½

5 medium tomatoes, chopped	¼ teaspoon garlic powder
2 stalks celery, chopped	½ teaspoon salt
2 medium carrots, chopped	½ teaspoon pepper
1 medium onion, chopped	½ teaspoon oregano
6 to 8 green onions, chopped	1 tablespoon vegetable or salad
1 packet Equal	oil
1 teaspoon basil	1 pound spaghetti

Put the vegetables in a pot and cover tightly. Cook over medium heat, stirring occasionally, for 10 minutes. Add the seasonings. Re-cover the pot and cook over medium-low heat for

˙ minutes. Add the oil and simmer for 30 minutes or until the carrots are tender. Cook the spaghetti. Drain. Toss with the sauce.

Stir-Fried Rice
(Serves 4)

With vegetables:
Calories per serving: 150
Fat per serving: $\frac{2}{5}$

With meat:
Calories per serving: 250 (approx.)
Fats per serving: $1\frac{2}{5}$ (approx.)

1 onion, chopped	1 to 2 large tomatoes, chopped
1 green pepper, chopped	1 cup any and all leftovers
2 cloves garlic, pressed	(vegetables or meat)
⅓ cup beef or chicken bouillon	2 tablespoons soy sauce
2 cups cooked brown rice	1 egg (optional)

Stir-fry the onion, pepper, and garlic in the bouillon until tender. Add all the other ingredients except the egg. Cook until hot. Add a beaten egg, if desired, and stir until the egg is cooked.

Birthday coming up?

Treat yourself to a new set of nonstick cookware — a must in low-fat cooking. In the meantime, invest in one of the commercial nonstick spray coatings for your pots and pans. These sprays are usually made from vegetable oils, and the amount you use makes a negligible addition to your daily fat intake. They save you hours of scrubbing — a real blessing.

Spanish Rice and Garbanzos
(Serves 6)

Calories per serving: 225
Fat per serving: ½

⅔ cup brown rice
1 small onion, chopped
⅓ cup chopped green pepper
¼ teaspoon garlic powder
1 teaspoon margarine
1 ½ cups water
½ teaspoon salt

¼ teaspoon pepper
1 16-ounce can tomatoes,
  broken up
1 15-ounce can garbanzos (or
  kidney beans), drained
½ teaspoon oregano

Sauté the rice, onion, green pepper, and garlic powder in the margarine, stirring occasionally, in a 2-quart saucepan over medium heat for about 5 minutes. Add the water, salt, and pepper. Bring to a boil. Reduce the heat, cover, and cook for 45 minutes or until the rice is tender and the liquid is absorbed. Stir in the tomatoes, garbanzos, and oregano. Cook for 5 minutes or until the mixture is heated through and the liquid is absorbed.

For fluffy rice:

Do not lift the lid or stir the rice while it cooks, or the grains will stick together. When the rice is done, remove the lid and cover the pot with two layers of paper toweling. Then cover with a tight-fitting lid and let stand 5 to 30 minutes or until you are ready to serve it. The excess moisture from the rice will be absorbed by the towels.

Rice-Stuffed Zucchini
(Serves 6)

Calories per serving: 153
Fat per serving: ⅕

4 medium zucchini	½ teaspoon basil
1 small onion, chopped	Salt and pepper to taste
1 teaspoon margarine	2¼ cups water
1 cup brown rice	2½ teaspoons chicken bouillon
3 tablespoons tomato paste	powder

Parboil the zucchini until just tender. Cut them in half length-wise and scrape out the seeds. Sauté the onion in the margarine until tender. Stir in the rice, tomato paste, basil, salt, pepper, water, and bouillon powder. Bring to a boil. Reduce the heat, cover, and simmer until the rice is tender and the liquid is absorbed. Cool. Spoon into the zucchini shells and bake at 350° for 20 minutes.

Rice Casserole
(Serves 4)

Calories per serving: 143
Fat per serving: ⅕

½ cup chopped celery	1 4-ounce can mushrooms,
½ cup chopped onion	drained
½ teaspoon margarine	2 teaspoons chicken bouillon
¾ cup brown rice	powder
2 cups boiling water	

Sauté the celery and onions in the margarine. Combine all the ingredients in a 2-quart casserole. Cover and bake at 350° for 1¼ hours or until the rice has absorbed the water.

Brown Rice Español
(Serves 6)

Calories per serving: 130
Fat per serving: $\frac{1}{10}$

1 16-ounce can tomatoes, cut
  up
1½ cups boiling water
1 teaspoon chicken bouillon
  powder
¾ cup chopped onion

1 tablespoon chopped jalapeño
  pepper
½ teaspoon garlic salt
2 teaspoons chili powder
1 cup uncooked brown rice

Bring the tomatoes, water, and bouillon powder to a boil. Stir
the remaining ingredients together in a 2-quart casserole. Add
the boiling tomato mixture and stir well. Cover tightly and
bake at 350° for 1¼ hours.

Brown and Wild Rice Pilaf
(Serves 10)

Calories per serving: 190
Fat per serving: $\frac{1}{5}$

2 cups brown rice
½ cup diced onion
1 teaspoon thyme

1 teaspoon black pepper
Pinch salt
4 cups chicken stock

Add the rice, onion, and seasonings to the stock and stir to coat
well. Bring to a simmer, cover, and cook until the liquid is absorbed and the rice is cooked.

¼ cup wild rice   ½ cup chicken stock

Add the rice to the stock. Bring to a simmer. Cover and cook
until the liquid is absorbed and the rice is cooked. Combine it
with the brown rice.

Risi e Bisi (Italian Rice and Peas)
(Serves 4)

Calories per serving: 160
Fat per serving: ⅕

2 cups hot, firmly cooked brown
  rice
1 cup boiling water
2 envelopes instant chicken
  broth and seasoning mix
1 teaspoon dehydrated onion
  flakes

2 teaspoons minced parsley
Pepper
Few drops sherry extract
¼ teaspoon margarine
1 16-ounce package frozen
  green peas

Combine all the ingredients in a small saucepan. Bring to a boil, reduce the heat, and simmer, covered, for 15 minutes or until the peas are soft. Remove the cover and continue to simmer if the peas and rice are too moist.

When cooking rice and other pasta, use chicken or vegetable stock or tomato juice instead of water.

Don't throw away leftover rice and grains. They can be reheated by simply adding 2 to 3 tablespoons of water to each cup of grain and simmering. Better yet, toss them into soups, stews, and salads.

Vegetables

Neapolitan Peas and Eggs
(Serves 5)

Calories per serving: 213
Fats per serving: 1⅘

¼ cup chopped onion
1 teaspoon vegetable oil
2 8-ounce cans tomato sauce
½ cup water

1 20-ounce bag frozen peas
¼ teaspoon pepper
5 eggs

Sauté the onion in the oil in a large skillet until tender. Add the tomato sauce and water and bring to a boil. Add the peas and pepper. Cook over high heat until the peas have thawed and separated. Lower the heat. Break the eggs carefully, one at a time, onto the pea mixture, far enough apart so they will cook separately. Cover tightly; simmer for 5 to 10 minutes or until the eggs are cooked to desired doneness.

What about eggs?

If your overall diet is low in fat and you don't have a cholesterol problem, by all means use eggs in moderation — 2 to 3 a week. They contain the highest quality protein you can find.

Eggplant Casserole
(Serves 6)

Calories per serving: 93
Fat per serving: $2/5$

1 eggplant, peeled and cut into
  thick chunks
4 tomatoes, peeled and cut into
  quarters
1 green pepper, diced
1 yellow squash, diced

1 onion, diced
1 teaspoon celery salt
1 teaspoon brown sugar
⅛ teaspoon garlic powder
5 slices Lite-line cheese

Combine all the ingredients, except the cheese, in a 2-quart nonstick casserole. Bake, covered, at 400° for 45 minutes to 1 hour or until the vegetables are tender. Arrange the slices of cheese on the top of the casserole, return to the oven, and bake for 5 minutes more.

Garden Casserole
(Serves 6)

Calories per serving: 117
Fat per serving: $1/5$

4 medium potatoes, peeled and
  sliced
1 onion, sliced
1 medium zucchini, sliced
2 carrots, pared and sliced
2 tomatoes, cut into small
  chunks

1 cup water
1 teaspoon chicken bouillon
  powder
¼ teaspoon pepper
1 teaspoon dill weed
Corn flake crumbs
3 slices Lite-line cheese

Spread the potatoes over the bottom of a 2-quart casserole. Separate the onions into rings and place them over the potatoes. Top these with the zucchini, then the carrots, and then the tomatoes. Heat the water and dissolve the bouillon powder in it. Add the pepper and dill weed. Pour over the casserole. Cover and bake at 375° for 1 hour. Sprinkle the crumbs over the top and arrange the slices of cheese over this. Return to the oven and bake for another 15 minutes.

Original recipe:

¼ cup butter instead of chicken bouillon
2 cups cheddar cheese instead of Lite-line
1 cup white wine instead of water

Calories per serving: 265
Fats per serving: 3

Swedish Green Beans
(Serves 6)

Calories per serving: 31
Fat per serving: trace

1 16-ounce can cut green beans
1 tablespoon chicken bouillon powder
3 tablespoons vinegar
1½ teaspoons sugar
Dash pepper
1 tablespoon cornstarch
1 tablespoon cold water
2 cups chopped cabbage (about ½ medium head)

Drain the liquid from the beans, add the next four ingredients to it, and heat to boiling, stirring. Stir in the cornstarch mixed with the water. Cook and stir until the mixture thickens and is clear. Add the cabbage and heat to boiling. Simmer, covered, for 35 minutes. Add the drained beans. Cook until hot.

How can you eat baked potatoes without butter and sour cream??
Try the following two recipes . . .

Baked Potato with Yogurt Topping
(Serves 4)

Calories per potato: 125
Fat per potato: trace

1 cup plain nonfat yogurt
1 tablespoon sesame seeds,
   toasted
Dill weed to taste
1 to 2 tablespoons Dijon mustard

2 tablespoons chopped green
   onions or chives
4 baked potatoes

Mix all the ingredients, except the potatoes, together. There
should be enough for a generous topping on each potato.

> This topping is also good on baked fish. Just spread
> it over the fish and follow baking directions.

Baked Potatoes with Beans

Calories per potato and topping: 235
Fat per potato and topping: 3/5

Cut a baked potato in half and push from both ends to make it
flaky. Place 2 tablespoons of low-fat cottage cheese on each
half. Add ¼ cup ranch-style beans (canned or homemade) over
the cottage cheese. Sprinkle with ½ ounce grated mozzarella

cheese and chopped green onions. Bake in a microwave, conventional, or toaster oven until the cheese melts.

P.S. Check our Sauces, Dips, and Dressings for other great potato toppings.

Baked potato with 1 tablespoon butter and 2 tablespoons sour cream:

Calories per potato and topping: 258
Fats per potato and topping: 3½

Potato-Cheese Soufflé
(Serves 4)

If you're in a hurry, you can use instant mashed potatoes in this recipe.

Calories per serving: 109
Fat per serving: ⅘

2 cups mashed potatoes, prepared with skim milk, no butter
2 eggs, slightly beaten

4 slices Lite-line cheese
¼ teaspoon pepper
¼ teaspoon garlic powder
Paprika

The mashed potatoes should have a soft consistency. If they are too thick, add a little skim milk. Beat in the eggs. Break up the cheese and beat into the potato mixture. Add the pepper and garlic powder and beat. Turn into a 1-quart nonstick casserole or pan. Sprinkle with paprika. Bake at 375° for 25 to 30 minutes until golden, puffed, and set. Serve at once.

Broccoli Neapolitan
(Serves 6)

Calories per serving: 68
Fat per serving: ½

2 teaspoons vegetable oil
½ cup chopped onion
½ teaspoon garlic salt
2 teaspoons flour
½ cup water
1 pound fresh broccoli, cut into florets

1 large carrot, cut into small pieces
2 medium tomatoes, chopped
½ teaspoon basil
½ teaspoon oregano
3 slices Lite-line cheese

Heat the oil in a skillet. Add the onion and garlic salt and stir until the onion is tender. Blend in the flour, stir in the water, and cook for 2 minutes. Add all the ingredients except the cheese. Stir, reduce the heat, and cover. Cook over low heat for about 20 minutes or until the broccoli and carrots are tender. Arrange the cheese slices on top and heat for a few minutes longer.

Spinach-Cheese Squares
(Serves 6)

Calories per serving: 112
Fat per serving: ⅗

1 tablespoon chopped onion
2 cups skim milk
2 tablespoons cornstarch
5 slices Lite-line cheese
2 eggs, slightly beaten

2 10-ounce packages frozen chopped spinach, cooked and drained
½ teaspoon salt
¼ teaspoon pepper

Cook the onion in a nonstick pan until soft. Add 1½ cups of the milk and heat. Mix the cornstarch with the remaining ½ cup of milk and add to the hot mixture, stirring until thick and smooth. Break up the cheese and add it. Slowly add the hot sauce to the beaten eggs, stirring constantly. Add the spinach, season with salt and pepper, and mix. Pour into an 8-inch-square oven dish and set it in a shallow pan of hot water. Bake at 350° for 45 minutes or until firm.

Original recipe:

Whole milk instead of skim
1 cup cheddar cheese instead of Lite-line
4 tablespoons butter

Calories per serving: 256
Fats per serving: $3\frac{2}{5}$

Spicy Green Beans
(Serves 4)

Calories per serving: 88
Fat per serving: $\frac{1}{5}$

1 medium onion, chopped	12 ounces beer
1 teaspoon margarine	1 pound green beans (fresh or
¼ teaspoon garlic powder	frozen, cut into 2-inch
¼ teaspoon dill weed	lengths)
⅛ teaspoon hot pepper flakes	½ cup chopped parsley
⅛ teaspoon salt	

Sauté the onion in the margarine for about 5 minutes. Add the herbs, spices, and beer. Bring to a boil and boil briskly for 3 minutes. Add the beans and cook, uncovered, for about 15 to 20 minutes or until the liquid has almost evaporated. Sprinkle with parsley and serve.

Fried Cabbage
(Serves 6)

Calories per serving: 42
Fat per serving: ⅗

1 large head cabbage, coarsely chopped	1 egg
	1 tablespoon skim milk
2 teaspoons bacon fat	2 tablespoons vinegar

Place the cabbage in a large bowl and cover with cold water. Let stand at least 1 hour. Drain, but don't shake off all the water. Heat the bacon fat in a large skillet and add the cabbage. Cover and cook over medium heat for about 20 minutes or until the cabbage is tender. Stir occasionally. Make a dressing of the egg, milk, and vinegar and pour it over the cabbage. Heat through, stirring often.

Spinach Soufflé
(Serves 6)

Calories per serving: 76
Fat per serving: ½

2 10-ounce packages frozen chopped spinach	3 eggs, separated
	1 medium onion, finely chopped
2 tablespoons cornstarch	1 tablespoon lemon juice
¼ cup skim milk	Salt and pepper to taste

Cook and drain the spinach. Dissolve the cornstarch in the milk. Beat the egg yolks and add to the cornstarch and milk. Stir this mixture into the spinach. Add the onion, lemon juice, and seasonings. Beat the egg whites until stiff. Fold them into the spinach mixture. Pour into a nonstick baking dish, place it in a pan of hot water, and bake at 350° for 30 to 45 minutes or until a knife inserted in the middle comes out clean.

Spinach-Artichoke Casserole
(Serves 6)

Calories per serving: 40
Fat per serving: $^1/_{10}$

2 10-ounce packages frozen
  chopped spinach
1 can water-packed artichoke
  hearts, chopped

½ cup low-fat cottage cheese
Salt and pepper to taste
Corn flake crumbs

Cook the spinach according to the directions. Drain well. Add the artichokes, cottage cheese, salt, and pepper. Top with the corn flake crumbs. Place in an 8-inch-square casserole and bake at 300° for about 20 to 30 minutes or until thoroughly heated.

Just Plain Steamed Vegetables

Calories per serving: 40
Fat per serving: trace

Select any fresh vegetables and wash them well. Trim and scrape them as needed, but do not peel them unless necessary. Fill a saucepan with about 1 inch of water. Place the vegetables in a steamer rack and lower the rack into the pan. (The water should not touch the vegetables.) Bring the water to a boil, cover, and reduce the heat. Steam until the vegetables are crisp and tender. Cooking time varies with the size and type of vegetable.

Serve with lemon juice and herbs or with one of our sauces in the Sauces, Dips, and Dressings section.

Vegetables are also delicious when steamed in a microwave oven. But models vary, so consult your instruction book for cooking times.

Breads

Oat-Wheat Bread
(Makes 4 loaves, 20 slices per loaf)

Calories per slice: 78
Fat per slice: 1/5

4 tablespoons margarine
5 teaspoons salt
2½ cups uncooked oatmeal
½ cup powdered milk
¾ cup molasses

4½ cups boiling water
2 packages active dry yeast
4½ cups stone-ground whole-wheat flour
6 cups unbleached white flour

Place the margarine, salt, oatmeal, powdered milk, and most of the molasses in a large bowl. Add 4 cups of the boiling water and stir until the margarine has melted. Add the yeast to the remaining ½ cup of cooled water (105–155°) to which a small amount of the molasses has been added. Add the yeast mixture to the oatmeal mixture. Stir in the whole-wheat and white flours. Add the flour until the dough is no longer sticky. Cover the dough with a towel. Let it rise until it doubles in bulk. Knead the dough and shape it into loaves. Place in lightly greased or nonstick bread pans. Cover the pans and let the dough rise again until it doubles in bulk. Bake at 375° for about 40 minutes. Remove the loaves from the pans immediately and place them on a rack to cool.

Easy Whole-Wheat Bread
(Makes 1 loaf, 20 slices)

Calories per slice: 110
Fats per slice: trace

2 cups whole-wheat flour
1 cup white flour
2 teaspoons baking soda
½ teaspoon salt

1 cup raisins
2 cups buttermilk (made from
   skim)
½ cup molasses

Mix the dry ingredients. Stir in the milk and molasses and mix thoroughly. Pour into a bread pan; let stand for 1 hour. Bake at 325° for about 1 hour or until done.

In baking use no more than ¼ cup sugar of any kind for each cup flour.

Applesauce Tea Bread
(Makes 1 loaf, 20 slices)

Calories per slice: 77
Fat per slice: $\frac{1}{10}$

2½ cups white flour
2 teaspoons baking powder
½ teaspoon salt
½ cup sugar

1 tablespoon cinnamon
8 ounces applesauce
1 egg
1 cup skim milk

Mix the dry ingredients together and add the applesauce, then the egg and milk. Pour into a nonstick loaf pan and bake at 350° for about 50 minutes. Remove the loaf from the pan and cool on a rack.

Prune Loaf
(Makes 1 loaf, 20 slices)

Without nuts:
Calories per slice: 78
Fat per slice: $\frac{1}{5}$

With nuts:
Calories per slice: 95
Fat per slice: $\frac{3}{5}$

1 cup boiling water
1 cup snipped pitted prunes
¾ cup whole-wheat flour
¼ cup white flour
1 teaspoon baking powder
½ teaspoon baking soda

½ teaspoon salt
1 cup wheat germ
1 egg
⅓ cup dark brown sugar
½ cup chopped walnuts
(optional)

Pour the water over the prunes. Stir the dry ingredients together and combine them with the prunes. Beat the egg with the sugar and add to the mixture, stirring until it is moist. Stir in the nuts. Bake in a nonstick loaf pan at 350° for 50 to 55 minutes. Remove the loaf from the pan and cool on a rack.

In baking, limit the amount of fat to 1 to 2 tablespoons per cup of whole-grain flour.

As a general rule of thumb in baking — Half the white flour in a recipe can be replaced with whole-wheat flour. Example: If a recipe calls for 2 cups white flour, use 1 cup white flour and 1 cup whole-wheat flour. The conversions have already been made in our recipes.

Bran Muffins
(Makes 12)

Without raisins:
Calories per muffin: 90
Fat per muffin: trace

With raisins:
Calories per muffin: 123
Fat per muffin: trace

1 cup white flour
2 cups bran
¼ cup cornmeal
1 teaspoon salt
1¼ cups skim milk

½ cup molasses
1 teaspoon baking soda dissolved in a little water
1 cup raisins (optional)

Mix all the ingredients together and pour into a muffin tin, using either a nonstick pan or paper liners. Bake at 325° for about 25 minutes.

Pineapple-Bran Whole-Wheat Muffins
(Makes 12)

Calories per muffin: 100
Fat per muffin: 1

1 cup whole-wheat flour
1 tablespoon baking powder
¼ teaspoon salt
1½ tablespoons brown sugar
1 egg
1 cup 100% all-bran cereal

⅓ cup skim milk
¼ cup vegetable oil
1 8-ounce can crushed pineapple (packed in unsweetened juice), undrained

Mix the flour, baking powder, salt, and sugar. Beat the egg slightly. Add the cereal, milk, and oil to the egg. Stir to combine. Let stand for 2 minutes or until the cereal has softened.

Stir the pineapple, including the juice, into the mixture. Add the flour mixture, stirring only until combined. Spoon the batter evenly into a paper-lined muffin tin and bake at 400° for about 25 minutes. Serve warm.

In baking you can usually cut the amount of salt in half with no noticeable difference in flavor.

Carrot or Zucchini Muffins
(Makes 24)

Calories per muffin: 88
Fat per muffin: 3/5

1½ cups whole-wheat flour
1 teaspoon salt
1½ teaspoons baking soda
1 teaspoon cinnamon
½ teaspoon nutmeg
1½ cups natural bran
3 medium carrots, cut into
   1-inch pieces (1 cup
   grated)—or use zucchini

2 eggs
¼ cup vegetable oil
1½ cups skim milk or orange
   juice
2 tablespoons vinegar
½ cup honey
¼ cup molasses
½ cup raisins

Blend the flour, salt, baking soda, cinnamon, nutmeg, and bran together in a food processor with a steel blade for 4 to 5 seconds. Pour into a large mixing bowl. Process the carrots until puréed and add to the dry ingredients. Process the eggs and oil for 2 to 3 seconds and add to the bowl along with the milk, vinegar, honey, molasses, and raisins. Stir with a wooden spoon until just blended; do not overmix. Spoon the batter into paper-lined muffin tins and bake at 375° for 20 to 25 minutes.

Whole-Wheat Carrot Muffins
(Makes 12)

Calories per muffin: 95
Fat per muffin: ½

1 ¼ cups whole-wheat flour
¼ cup all-purpose flour
2 teaspoons baking powder
¼ teaspoon salt
2 eggs

1 cup plain low-fat yogurt
2 tablespoons molasses
1 tablespoon vegetable oil
½ cup shredded carrots

Stir together the flours, baking powder, and salt in a large bowl; beat the eggs with a fork in a small bowl; beat in the yogurt, molasses, and oil; stir in the carrots. Add to the flour mixture and stir until just moistened. Spoon the batter into a paper-lined muffin tin. Bake at 375° for 15 to 20 minutes. Serve warm.

Banana-Raisin Muffins
(Makes 12)

Calories per muffin: 160
Fat per muffin: ⅕

2 cups whole-wheat flour
1 cup unprocessed bran flakes
1 cup rolled oats
1 ½ teaspoons baking soda
2 egg whites

¾ cup frozen apple juice concentrate, thawed
½ cup plain low-fat yogurt
1 cup mashed bananas
1 cup raisins

Combine the flour, bran flakes, rolled oats, and baking soda in a large bowl. Beat the egg whites in a small bowl until stiff peaks form, and set aside. Add the apple juice, yogurt, bananas, and raisins to the flour mixture and stir to blend. Fold in the egg whites and mix well. Spoon the batter into a paper-lined muffin tin and bake at 400° for 20 minutes.

Whole-Wheat Buckys
(Makes 12)

Calories per pancake: 88
Fat per pancake: $3/5$

1 egg
1 tablespoon honey
1 ½ cups buttermilk (made from
   skim)
2 tablespoons vegetable oil

1 cup buckwheat flour
½ cup whole-wheat flour
2 teaspoons baking powder
1 teaspoon baking soda
½ teaspoon salt

Beat the egg, honey, buttermilk, and oil together. Thoroughly blend in the dry ingredients. Drop by spoonfuls onto a lightly oiled skillet and bake, browning on both sides.

Mock Soufflé
(Serves 4)

We've enjoyed this soufflé for breakfast many times. At breakfast add a bowl of fresh fruit; at lunch, a mixed salad.

Calories per serving: 145
Fat per serving: 1

3 slices whole-wheat bread,
   crusts removed and cut into
   small cubes
4 slices Lite-line cheese, torn up
2 eggs

¼ teaspoon salt
½ teaspoon dry mustard
Pepper
1 ⅓ cups skim milk

Mix the bread and cheese. Beat the eggs; add the seasonings and milk. Add to the bread and cheese. Chill overnight. Bake in a 1-quart casserole set in a pan of hot water at 350° for 1¼ hours.

Calzone with Zucchini Filling
(Makes 6)

Calories per piece: 283
Fats per piece: 1 ⅕

1 ½ teaspoons active dry yeast	1 ½ cups whole-wheat flour
1 cup warm water (105–115°)	1 ½ cups whole-wheat pastry
1 teaspoon sugar	flour
1 ½ teaspoons salt	Zucchini filling (see below)

Coat a cookie sheet with nonstick vegetable spray and set aside. Sprinkle the yeast over the warm water in a large bowl; let stand for 5 minutes. Stir in the sugar and salt. Stir the flours together in a separate bowl until blended. Add 2½ cups of the flour to the yeast. Knead with the remaining flour, as necessary, for 10 to 15 minutes, until the dough is smooth and elastic. Place the dough in a bowl, cover, and let rise in a warm place until it doubles in bulk — about 1 hour. While the dough is rising, make the filling. Punch down the dough, divide it into 6 pieces, and roll them out into ¼-inch-thick rounds. Spoon ⅓ cup of the filling on one-half of each circle, leaving a half-inch rim. Moisten the edges with water, fold over, and seal the edges with a fork. Prick the dough in several places. Place on the cookie sheet and bake at 450° for 15 minutes or until lightly browned.

Zucchini Filling

½ cup minced onion	½ cup crumbled feta cheese
2 small cloves garlic, crushed	½ cup grated Swiss cheese
2 medium zucchini, sliced	¾ teaspoon dill weed
1 large tomato, chopped	¾ teaspoon salt
1 egg	⅛ teaspoon pepper

Sauté the onion and garlic in a nonstick skillet until tender. Add the zucchini and tomato. Cover and cook for 5 to 6 minutes or until the zucchini is tender-crisp. Place the zucchini mixture in a bowl and add the egg, cheeses, dill weed, salt, and pepper; mix well.

Apple Stuffing
(Serves 6)

Calories per serving: 200
Fat per serving: ½

12 slices whole-wheat bread,
   cut into ½-inch cubes
½ cup chopped onion
½ cup chopped celery
1 tablespoon chopped parsley
⅛ teaspoon salt

⅛ teaspoon pepper
1½ cups skim milk
1 egg, lightly beaten
2 medium apples, pared, cored,
   and chopped
¼ cup raisins (optional)

Bake the bread cubes on a cookie sheet at 375° for about 5 minutes. Put the cubes in a large bowl. Cook the onion, celery, parsley, salt, and pepper in a small amount of water for about 5 minutes. Pour over the bread. Add the milk and egg and stir. Gently stir in the apples, and the raisins if desired. Spoon into a 2-quart nonstick baking dish and bake at 350° for 1 hour.

In baking:

- Substitute 1 6-ounce can unsweetened frozen fruit juice concentrate for ½ cup sugar. (Decrease the liquid by 2 tablespoons and add a pinch of baking soda unless yogurt, buttermilk, or sour milk is used in the recipe.)
- Substitute ¼ cup applesauce or fruit juice and ¼ cup butter or oil for ½ cup shortening.
- In recipes that specify 2 eggs you can substitute 1 whole egg and 2 egg whites, reducing the calories from 156 to 95 and the fats from 2 to 1.

Quick French Toast
(Serves 4)

Calories per serving: 90
Fat per serving: ⅕

½ cup skim milk   ½ cup fruit-flavored low-fat
4 egg whites   yogurt
4 slices whole-wheat bread

Mix the milk and egg whites. Coat the bread with the mixture
and cook in a nonstick pan over medium heat, turning once,
until both sides are golden brown. Top with the yogurt.

Toppings for pancakes, waffles, and french toast:

- Fresh or frozen fruit blended until mushy
- Fresh or frozen fruit blended with plain low-fat
  yogurt
- Fruit-flavored low-fat yogurt

Desserts

Apple Cake for C.B.
(Serves 8)

When my son, the author-lecturer, was growing up, he ran a lot and exercised diligently. So I could use this recipe (one of his favorites) with no hesitation despite its slightly high fat content. He said I could insert it in his cookbook if you readers who don't run or exercise would promise not to use it. — Covert's Mom

Calories per serving: 295
Fats per serving: $2\frac{1}{5}$

⅓ cup margarine
⅔ cup sugar
1 cup white flour
1 cup whole-wheat flour
½ teaspoon cinnamon
½ teaspoon ground cloves
½ teaspoon nutmeg

½ teaspoon salt
1 teaspoon baking soda dissolved in ⅔ cup water
1 cup finely chopped apple
⅓ cup raisins
⅓ cup chopped walnuts
2 egg whites, whipped

Cream the margarine and sugar. Add the dry ingredients and water alternately, then the apple. Dust the raisins and nuts with a small amount of flour and add them to the batter. Fold in the egg whites. Bake in an 8-inch-square nonstick pan at 350° for 30 to 40 minutes or until firm.

P.S. We must confess to modifying Mom's recipe; her original had 1 whole egg, 1 cup sugar, ½ cup butter, and white flour only, yielding 369 calories and $3\frac{1}{5}$ fats per serving.

Baked Apple Meringue with Custard Sauce
(Serves 4)

This is a delicious and attractive dessert.

Calories per serving: 105
Fat per serving: ⅗

2 medium cooking apples, cored and halved crosswise	2 egg whites
½ cup water	¼ teaspoon cream of tartar
¾ teaspoon cinnamon	1 packet Equal

Place the apples, cut sides up, in a shallow baking dish and add the water. Sprinkle with the cinnamon. Bake at 350° for about 25 minutes or until tender. Remove from the oven. Beat the egg whites and cream of tartar until stiff. Beat in the Equal. Spoon onto the apples, forming peaks. Bake at 200° for 5 to 7 minutes or until the meringue is lightly browned. Serve with Custard Sauce.

Custard Sauce

2 egg yolks, lightly beaten	½ teaspoon vanilla
1 cup skim milk	2 teaspoons rum flavoring
1 packet Equal	Nutmeg

Mix the egg yolks, milk, Equal, and vanilla well. Cook over medium-low heat, stirring constantly, for 3 to 5 minutes or until the mixture thickly coats a metal spoon. Remove from the heat. Stir in the rum flavoring. Strain into a bowl. Cover and chill. Serve over the apple meringues. Sprinkle with nutmeg.

Blueberry Bread Pudding
(Serves 6 to 8)

Calories per serving: 140
Fat per serving: ½

3 tablespoons sugar
¼ teaspoon salt
½ teaspoon vanilla
2 eggs, beaten
½ teaspoon almond extract

2½ to 3 cups whole-wheat
    bread, cubed
¾ cup skim milk, scalded
2 cups frozen blueberries,
    thawed

Combine the sugar, salt, vanilla, eggs, and almond extract. Add the bread cubes and mix well. Slowly add the milk, stirring constantly. Add the berries. Pour into a 2-quart nonstick (or lightly greased) casserole, set in a pan of hot water, and bake at 350° for 1 hour. Serve warm.

Lemony Baked Apples
(Serves 4)

Very tart!

Calories per serving: 242
Fat per serving: ⅕

4 large Delicious apples, cored
1 6-ounce can frozen lemonade
    concentrate, thawed

4 teaspoons brown sugar

Peel the apples a third of the way down from the stem. Arrange them in a shallow baking dish. Spoon the lemonade into the cavities and over the tops of the apples. Sprinkle with the brown sugar. Bake at 350°, basting occasionally, for about 1 hour or until the apples are tender but retain their shape. Serve warm or at room temperature.

Quick Sherbet
(Serves 4)

Calories per serving: 50
Fat per serving: trace

1 16-ounce can mixed fruit (or
   sliced peaches or pears),
   packed in juice or extra-light
   syrup

Freeze the can until solid. Place it under hot water for 1 minute. Open the can, put the fruit in a blender, and process until it is the consistency of sherbet. If necessary, return it to the freezer until serving time. Serve plain or over melon slices.

Buttermilk Sherbet
(Serves 6)

I'm not fond of either buttermilk or pineapple, so this recipe sounded terrible. But was I surprised . . . !! — C.B.

Calories per serving: 90
Fat per serving: trace

2 cups buttermilk (made from   1 egg white
   skim)   1 ½ teaspoons vanilla
½ cup sugar
1 cup crushed pineapple,
   drained

Combine the buttermilk, sugar, and pineapple and freeze the mixture until it has a mushy consistency. Place it in a chilled bowl and add the egg white and vanilla. Beat the sherbet until it is light and fluffy. Replace it in the refrigerator tray and freeze until it is firm, stirring frequently.

Frozen Raspberry Yogurt
(Serves 4)

Calories per serving: 211
Fat per serving: ½

1 pint fresh or thawed frozen
loose-pack raspberries (or
blackberries)

2 cups plain low-fat yogurt
½ cup granulated sugar
½ teaspoon vanilla

Purée the berries in a blender until almost smooth. Strain them to remove the seeds and set aside. Mix the yogurt, sugar, and vanilla until smooth. Stir into the puréed berries until well blended. Churn in an ice cream maker for about 10 to 15 minutes or until frozen. If you use blackberries, you don't have to strain them; just mix all the ingredients together in the blender.

Lime Chiffon Pudding
(Serves 8)

Calories per serving: 114
Fat per serving: ½

1 envelope unflavored gelatin
½ cup cold water
⅛ teaspoon salt

4 eggs, separated
1 6-ounce can frozen limeade
⅓ cup sugar

Sprinkle the gelatin over the cold water in a medium-sized saucepan. Add the salt and egg yolks; mix well. Place over low heat and cook, stirring constantly, for about 3 to 5 minutes or until the mixture thickens slightly and the gelatin dissolves. Remove from the heat and add the limeade; stir until melted. The mixture should mound slightly when dropped from a spoon. If it doesn't, chill it for a few minutes. Beat the egg whites until stiff, but not dry. Gradually add the sugar and beat until very stiff. Fold in the gelatin mixture. Mound in sherbet dishes. Chill until firm.

The next three recipes can also be used as pie fillings. But pie crust makes the fats go up awfully fast. One typical slice of crust (without the filling) contains 3 fats.

Orange Pudding
(Serves 6)

Calories per serving: 80
Fat per serving: ½

1 cup orange juice
1 teaspoon grated orange rind
1 tablespoon lemon juice

3 tablespoons flour
3 eggs, separated
10 packets Equal

Combine the orange juice, rind, lemon juice, flour, egg yolks, and Equal in a pan. Stir over low heat until thickened. Cool. Whip the egg whites until stiff, then fold them carefully into the cooled custard. Pour into dessert dishes and chill well for 12 hours.

Easy Chocolate Pudding for Children
(Serves 4)

With sugar:
Calories per serving: 208
Fat per serving: ⅕

With Sweet 'n Low:
Calories per serving: 160
Fat per serving ⅕

¼ cup sugar or 2 packets
 Sweet 'n Low
2 tablespoons cocoa
3 tablespoons cornstarch

Pinch salt
2 cups skim milk
1 teaspoon vanilla

Mix the dry ingredients. Add the milk and vanilla and cook until thickened. Refrigerate.

Low-Fat Berry Pudding
(Serves 4)

Calories per serving: 196
Fat per serving: ½

2 cups plain low-fat yogurt
1 3-ounce package instant vanilla pudding

1 ½ cups berries
3 packets Equal or sugar substitute

Combine the yogurt, pudding, berries, and Equal in a mixer.
Chill well.

Sugar or sugar substitutes?

Ideally, one should learn to eat well without relying
on sweeteners. But we admit it — we sometimes
get the craving, too. Personally, we are less ada-
mant about sugar restriction than about fat restriction. As noted in *Fit or Fat?,* fit people handle sugar
better than fat people. The fit individual tolerates the
occasional use of sucrose well. (Of course, you're
brushing and flossing afterward!) However, if you're
not fit and perhaps overfat, we recommend that you
use the sugar substitutes. The studies showing
cancer linkage with sugar substitutes are tentative
and vague at best. Massive quantities of sugar substitutes are necessary to produce cancer in rats.
The amount of any of the well-known substitutes
you would have to consume to endanger yourself is
far in excess of anything you would ordinarily use.
In any case, we consider the sugar substitutes to be
the lesser of two evils; that is, it's worth the minor
risk if it helps in any way to overcome obesity and all
its related medical problems.

Meringue Tarts with Strawberries
(Makes 8)

Calories per tart: 122
Fat per tart: trace

1 cup sugar
½ teaspoon baking powder
⅛ teaspoon salt
3 egg whites

1 teaspoon vanilla
1 teaspoon vinegar
1 teaspoon water
Fresh sliced strawberries

Sift the sugar with the baking powder and salt. Combine the liquids. Add the sugar, ½ teaspoon at a time, to the egg whites, alternating with a few drops of the liquid, beating constantly. When all the ingredients have been combined, continue to beat for several minutes. Place large spoonfuls on a baking sheet and shape into shallow cups. Bake at 225° for 45 minutes to 1 hour. Remove the meringues from the sheet quickly and cool them on a rack. Fill with strawberries.

Here are three custard recipes. The first is for people who can eat from Category 1, the second for Category 2, and the third for Category 3.

Covert's Coveted Custard
(Serves 8)

Calories per serving: 132
Fat per serving: 1

Category 1
4 eggs
⅓ cup sugar
½ teaspoon sal

1 quart 2% low-fat milk, scalded
1 teaspoon vanilla

Calories per serving: 100
Fat per serving: $\frac{2}{5}$

Category 2

2 eggs plus 2 egg whites	1 quart skim milk, scalded
⅓ cup sugar	1 teaspoon vanilla
½ teaspoon salt	

The cooking directions for both categories are the same. Beat the eggs slightly in a large mixing bowl; add the sugar and salt and beat to combine. Gradually and vigorously stir in the milk, then the vanilla. Put the mixture in eight 6-ounce custard cups and place the cups in a shallow roasting pan. Pour boiling water around the cups to almost the height of the custard. Bake in a preheated 350° oven for 30 minutes or until a silver knife inserted in the center comes out clean. Remove the cups from the water and cool on a wire rack. Cover and chill.

Custard with Egg Whites
(Serves 5)

Calories per serving: 87
Fat per serving: trace

Category 3

4 egg whites	¼ teaspoon almond extract
¼ cup sugar	½ teaspoon vanilla
2 cups skim milk, scalded	⅛ teaspoon nutmeg

Beat the egg whites until stiff. Gradually beat the sugar into the egg whites until well incorporated. Very gradually, but vigorously, add the milk to the egg mixture; then beat in the almond extract, vanilla, and nutmeg. Pour the mixture into custard cups. Place the cups in a shallow roasting pan. Pour boiling water around the cups to almost the height of the custard. Bake at 325° for about 1 hour. Remove the cups from the water and cool on a wire rack. Chill. Serve with puréed strawberries.

Rolled-Oat Macaroons
(Makes 36)

Calories per macaroon: 53
Fat per macaroon: $\frac{1}{5}$

2½ teaspoons melted butter
1 cup brown sugar, closely
  packed
2 eggs, separated

2½ cups rolled oats
2 teaspoons baking powder
1 teaspoon vanilla
⅛ teaspoon salt

Combine the butter, sugar, egg yolks, rolled oats, baking powder, and vanilla and beat well. Whip the egg whites until they are stiff and fold them and the salt into the other ingredients. Drop by teaspoonfuls, 3 inches apart, onto a nonstick cookie sheet. Bake at 375° for about 10 minutes.

Carrot-Oatmeal Cookies
(Makes 48)

Calories per cookie: 46
Fat per cookie: $\frac{1}{5}$

½ cup all-purpose flour
½ cup whole-wheat flour
¼ cup nonfat dry milk powder
1 teaspoon baking powder
¼ teaspoon baking soda
½ teaspoon salt
¼ teaspoon ground nutmeg
¼ teaspoon ground cinnamon

¼ cup solid shortening
⅓ cup brown sugar
½ cup molasses
1 egg
1 cup shredded carrots
1 teaspoon vanilla
1¾ cups quick-cooking rolled
  oats

Combine the flours, milk powder, baking powder, baking soda, salt, nutmeg, and cinnamon. Cream together the shortening, sugar, and molasses; add the egg, then the dry ingredients. Stir until well blended. Add the carrots, vanilla, and oats and mix well. Drop by teaspoonfuls onto an ungreased cookie sheet. Bake in a preheated 375° oven for 10 to 12 minutes or until lightly browned. Remove the cookies and cool on a wire rack.

Most cookies run about ½ fat each. So you can eat two and a half Rolled-Oat Macaroons or Carrot-Oatmeal Cookies for the price (fat) of one!

Scotch Apple Pudding
(Serves 6 to 8)

Yummy!

Calories per serving: 155
Fat per serving: ⅖

4 large apples, pared and cored   1 teaspoon butter
⅓ cup sugar   ½ cup rolled oats
⅛ teaspoon cinnamon   1½ cups skim milk
⅛ teaspoon salt

Cut the apples into slices. Combine the sugar, cinnamon, and salt. Place half the apples in a nonstick baking dish and sprinkle with half the sugar mixture. Dot with half the butter. Sprinkle half the oats over all. Arrange another series of layers. Then add the milk. Cover the dish and bake at 350° for 45 minutes. Remove the cover and bake for 15 minutes more. Serve hot or cold.

Snacks and
Beverages

Double Beanie
(Serves 2)

No. 1, calories per serving: 118
Fat per serving: $\frac{1}{5}$

No. 2, calories per serving: 105
Fat per serving: $\frac{1}{10}$

2 slices whole-wheat, rye, or
  pumpernickel bread
1 8-ounce can baked beans
2 tablespoons low-fat cottage
  cheese

Garlic salt
Paprika
½ small onion or 1 scallion,
  finely chopped
Chili powder

Beanie No. 1
Spread one slice of the bread with a generous layer of the beans. Add a covering of cottage cheese. Sprinkle with garlic salt to taste. Add a dash or two of paprika.

Beanie No. 2
Spread the beans on the second slice of bread as above. Cover generously with the onion. Add several dashes of chili powder.

Place both slices under the broiler until they are well warmed and slightly brown. Cut the slices in half and serve half of each piece to two people.

Tuna 'n' Cheese Snack
(Serves 4)

Calories per serving: 113
Fat per serving: $\frac{1}{5}$

4 slices whole-wheat or whole-   ½ cup low-fat cottage cheese
   rye bread   3 to 4 drops Tabasco sauce
½ cup water-packed tuna

Turn the oven to broil. Toast the bread under the broiler for 20 to 30 seconds on each side or until it is crisp. Mix the tuna, cottage cheese, and Tabasco sauce, and spread it on the toast. Return to the broiler for 20 to 30 seconds or until the cheese has melted.

Broiled Stuffed Mushroom Caps
(Serves 1)

Calories per serving: 44
Fat per serving: trace

4 medium-large mushrooms   1 teaspoon taco seasoning
2 tablespoons 100% all-bran
   cereal

Chop the stems of the mushrooms. Add the cereal and seasoning. Fill the caps and place them under a broiler for 4 to 5 minutes. Don't burn!

Apple-Flavored Yogurt
(Serves 2)

With low-fat yogurt:
Calories per serving: 120
Fat per serving: ½

With nonfat yogurt:
Calories per serving: 85
Fat per serving: trace

1 cup plain low-fat *or* nonfat
   yogurt
1 cup unsweetened applesauce
½ teaspoon cinnamon

1 packet Equal (optional)
2 to 3 teaspoons unprocessed
   bran

Combine the yogurt, applesauce, cinnamon, and Equal. Refrigerate for 2 hours. Add the bran just before serving and stir well.

Bananas Rhyder
(Serves 4)

Calories per serving: 160
Fat per serving: ⅕

2 bananas, peeled and frozen
2 pears, peeled, sliced, and frozen

1 apple, peeled, sliced, and frozen
½ cup plain low-fat yogurt

Slice the bananas. Place them and the remaining ingredients in a food processor or blender and purée. It is usually necessary to turn off the processor or blender every 30 seconds or so and mash down any lumps with a soft plastic spoon. Serve immediately.

Yogurt Fruitsicles
(Makes 6)

Calories per fruitsicle: 150
Fat per fruitsicle: ⅕

2 cups vanilla low-fat yogurt
1 6-ounce can frozen apple
   juice concentrate

¼ cup lemon or lime juice
2 cups any other unsweetened
   fruit juice

Combine the yogurt, apple juice, and lemon juice, then add the last fruit juice. Place the mixture in a blender and mix well. Pour into molds and freeze.

Strawberry Yogurt Frost
(Serves 3)

Calories per serving: 91
Fat per serving: ½

1 ¼ cups frozen strawberries *or*
   1 ½ cups fresh berries
⅓ cup instant nonfat dry milk
1 cup plain low-fat yogurt

¾ cup water
2 packets Equal
1 teaspoon vanilla

Place all the ingredients in a blender. Cover and process until smooth.

You can make nutritious drinks even if you don't have a blender. Simply mix up a quart of nonfat dry milk according to the directions on the package and store it in the refrigerator. Add flavoring and other ingredients as desired.

Arctic Fruit Frappe
(Makes 6 cups)

Calories per ½ cup: 70
Fat per ½ cup: trace

2 cups skim milk
1 cup nonfat dry milk
1 8-ounce can frozen unsweetened orange juice *or* pineapple juice *or* apple juice
concentrate

2 cups fresh strawberries *or*
fresh peaches *or* 1 cup unsweetened crushed pineapple

Mix the milks together. Add the fruit juice, then the fruit.
Blend well and freeze. Stir every 2 or 3 hours.

Nutmeg Nog
(Serves 1)

Calories per serving: 183
Fat per serving: 1

1 egg
1 teaspoon sugar
1 cup skim milk

¼ teaspoon vanilla
Nutmeg

Beat the egg until light and foamy. Add the sugar and beat
until thick and lemon-colored. Gradually mix in the milk and
vanilla. Pour into a glass and sprinkle with nutmeg.

Commercial egg nog:

Calories per cup: 342
Fats per cup: 4

Orange Cow
(Makes 4 cups)

Calories per cup: 105
Fat per cup: $1/5$

¾ cup cold water
1 egg
1 6-ounce can unsweetened frozen orange juice concentrate

½ cup instant nonfat dry milk
1 packet Equal
1 teaspoon vanilla
10 ice cubes

Place all the ingredients in a blender. Cover and process at high speed until smooth. Garnish with a slice of orange.

Hi-Fiber Lo-Fat Fruit Bran Milk Shake
(Makes 2 generous shakes)

Calories per shake: 180
Fat per shake: $1/5$

3 cups skim milk
¼ cup 100% all-bran cereal
¼ teaspoon cinnamon
¼ to ½ teaspoon vanilla

1 medium apple, cored, sec-
   tioned, and unpeeled *or*
   1 cup fresh strawberries *or*
   1 banana *or* 1 medium pear
   or peach

Freeze 2½ cups of the milk in a cube tray overnight. Put the bran, cinnamon, vanilla, and fruit into a blender. Add the remaining ½ cup of milk. Blend for 20 seconds. Continue blending and slowly, one at a time, add two-thirds of the frozen milk cubes. (Save the remaining cubes for future milk shakes.)

> A 2-cup regular homemade milk shake has 840 cal-
> ories and 7 fats.

Vanilla Delight
(Serves 1)

Calories per serving: 109
Fat per serving: trace

1 cup skim milk   1 teaspoon honey
½ teaspoon vanilla

Combine the ingredients in a tall glass and stir.

Don't let the word *natural* fool you. "Natural" foods can be loaded with fat and sugar. All the following are sweeteners and should not be considered "better" than sugar: sucrose, glucose, fructose, corn syrup, invert sugar, brown sugar, honey, and molasses.

Recommended
Low-Fat Cookbooks
Index

Recommended Low-Fat Cookbooks

Beautiful Food . . . for Your Beautiful Body by Jeanette Silveira Burke
>Send $11.00 (includes postage) to: Jeanette Burke, 1417 N. Birch, Reedley, CA 93654

This is the king of low-fat cookbooks! It not only has over 300 great recipes but serves as an excellent textbook for those who want to read more on the subject. Jeanette Burke teaches nutrition at a community college; her writing on the subject is a delight. The book is chock-full of suggestions and facts, making it a must for any cook's library.

The I Love to Eat but Hate to Diet Cookbook by Joan Mary Alimonti
>Send $8.50 (includes postage) to: Asta Productions, P.O. Box 3238, Walnut Creek, CA 94598

Joan Alimonti is our kind of writer. In fact, we liked the format of her book so well that we designed ours the same way. Her more than 270 recipes are simple, easy to follow, and low in fat and sugar. Each recipe is analyzed according to the diabetic exchange system. We especially enjoyed the Breakfasts section.

No Salt, No Sugar, No Fat Cookbook
  Send $7.00 (includes postage) to: Nitty Gritty Productions, P.O.
  Box 5457-NO, Concord, CA 94524

This is a fine little cookbook (120 recipes) with an excellent section
on legumes. The author has lots of ideas and hints on how to intro-
duce high fiber into the diet, along with ways to replace salt.

The Lowfat Lifestyle by Ronda Gates and Valerie Parker
  Send $8.50 (includes postage) to: Ronda Gates, P.O. Box 1843,
  Lake Oswego, OR 97035

The authors, using Covert Bailey's Target Diet system, analyze 200
low-fat recipes. This entertaining book also contains easy-to-read
information on nutrition, anecdotes about lifestyle changes, fitness
tips, and a section on exercise.

Lean Life Cuisine by Eve Lowry and Carla Mulligan
  Available in most bookstores; $4.50 (approx.)

Each recipe is analyzed for its fat, protein, carbohydrate, and fiber
content and is accompanied by a complete nutrient density graph.
Fats and sugars are reduced as much as possible without eliminat-
ing flavor.

The Live Longer Now Cookbook by Jon Leonard and Elaine Taylor
  Available in most bookstores; $3.50 (approx.)

This cookbook is based on the Pritikin Diet, which we feel is too
strict for the average person. Nonetheless, we recommend these recipes (over 300) for their creativity. If you enjoy cooking and have
the time, you'll discover many new ways to lower dietary fat (make
your own yogurt, sour cream, etc.) and cook high-fiber dishes.

Index